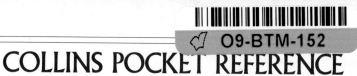

09-BTM-152

# COLLINS POCKET REFERENCE

# WOMEN'S HEALTH

Robert M. Youngson

HarperCollins*Publishers*

HarperCollins Publishers
P.O. Box, Glasgow G4 0NB

First published 1994

Reprint 10 9 8 7 6 5 4 3 2 1

© Robert M. Youngson 1994

ISBN 0 00 470539 4

A catalogue record for this book is available
from the British Library

Printed in Hong Kong

# INTRODUCTION

As a woman, you can congratulate yourself that, with any luck, you are likely to live quite a lot longer than the average man. This is quite remarkable, considering that women can suffer from many conditions that never affect men. A woman's body must be capable of the complex processes of childbearing and infant feeding. In addition, there are some disorders unconnected with the reproductive system that, for reasons not always clear, tend to affect women more than they affect men.

In planning this book I had to bear these facts in mind. I then had to select, from the large number of subjects that might have been included, those that I thought would be most useful and interesting to women. There are many conditions affecting both sexes that I would like to have dealt with. But I really had to confine the entries to those matters that affect women either exclusively or much more often than men.

There are so many important and worthwhile things I am anxious to tell you about women's health – things that can make a world of difference to you – that I am delighted to have this opportunity to write about many of them. My first aim has been to make the book useful and the information in it accessible. This is why I have arranged it in an A to Z format. I have also tried, whenever possible, to lead you into the section you need by including as many cross-references as possible. Words in small capital letters are cross references to other entries. Because every subject covered could have one of a number of possible headings, I had to settle for a fairly standard medical description and this may not be familiar to you. This is why these cross-references, however annoying, are necessary.

It is impossible for me to write a book of this kind without expressing personal bias. So as to minimize this I have had the benefit of critical reading of the whole manuscript by Dr Angela Railton, a distinguished consultant gynaecologist and obstetrician. I am deeply indebted to her for her pertinent comments, judicious amendments and most helpful suggestions. I am also most grateful to my tactful and cheerful editor at HarperCollins, Gail Strachan.

No book can ever be an adequate substitute for a proper medical consultation with a good and sympathetic doctor, but a little timely information can often relieve anxiety, help you to avoid danger or prompt you to take necessary action. Above all, knowledge about your body and about the things that can happen to it is an essential factor in helping you to achieve the highest possible level of good health – and a long life.

Dr Robert M. Youngson,
London 1994

# THE
# A TO Z
# OF
# WOMEN'S HEALTH

# A

### Abortion

This term means the loss of the fetus before it is able to survive outside the UTERUS. This applies both to spontaneous MIS-CARRIAGE and deliberate termination of pregnancy, either legally for medical reasons or as a criminal act. It is believed that as many as one in five pregnancies end in spontaneous miscarriage and that many of these are caused by a serious abnormality of the embryo or fetus.

Deliberate termination of pregnancy is called induced abortion. When this is legal it is called *therapeutic abortion*. If there are good reasons, abortion may be performed legally under certain circumstances and in approved hospitals or clinics. Two doctors, who have seen the patient, must agree that continuation of the pregnancy would be detrimental to her or her existing children's physical or mental health. The criteria are more relaxed in the USA. Following a Supreme Court decision in 1973, abortion under 12 weeks is permitted if the woman wishes it and her doctor agrees. Some States are reviewing this policy and a court ruling in 1989 has strengthened the position of the anti-abortion lobby.

Many abortions are done for 'social' or alleged psychiatric reasons, the remainder because of organic medical disorders. Some forms of heart or kidney disease and some cancers – especially those of the neck of the cervix or of the breast, may be made worse by pregnancy, and almost all doctors believe that abortion is justified in such cases. Certain abnormalities in the fetus, which would lead to an abnormal baby, are also considered to justify abortion. Many of these can be diagnosed by ultrasound scan, by AMNIOCENTESIS or by CHORIONIC VILLUS SAMPLING.

Therapeutic abortion is safest before 12 weeks and the method varies with the stage in pregnancy. General anaesthesia is almost always used. Up to about 14 weeks, abortion is commonly procured by dilatation of the cervix with a succession of smooth rods of increasing diameter, followed by vacuum suction through a tube or gentle scraping (*curettage*). The drug Mifepristone is now being widely used to terminate pregnancy up to about nine weeks.

After 14 weeks, medical methods are usual. Often, a hormone called a prostaglandin is used. When some of this is put into the uterus, it contracts down and the cervix widens, as in a normal delivery. The procedure is always done in hospital. A prostaglandin can also be injected into a vein but is more commonly given in a PESSARY, which melts after being placed in the VAGINA. The patient is given drugs to control the pain of the contractions and remains awake. The procedure usually takes about 12 hours. Sometimes expulsion of the fetus is incomplete and an ERPC (evacuation of retained products of conception) is necessary (see MISCARRIAGE), but usually the patient leaves hospital within 24 to 48 hours after the operation.

Criminal abortion is the termination or attempted termination of a pregnancy performed illegally or by unqualified persons. Many 'backstreet' abortionists have little idea of safe practice and there is a high risk of serious injury. This may be immediate, from perforation of the uterus, for instance, or from severe bleeding, or it may occur later from infection, often leading to permanent infertility.

## Absent menstruation
See AMENORRHOEA.

## Acne
See SKIN DISORDERS.

## Afterbirth
The placenta, the umbilical cord and the ruptured membranes which surrounded the fetus before birth. These parts are normally expelled from the UTERUS within an hour or two of birth.

## Afterpains
In returning to its normal size after childbirth, the UTERUS must undergo considerable contraction. This takes a few days, during which the mother may suffer pains similar to, but less severe than, those of labour. The pain may become more severe during breast feeding. Painkillers may be needed.

## AIDS
The Acquired Immune Deficiency Syndrome is caused by the human immunodeficiency virus (HIV), but this is not necessarily acquired by sexual transmission. HIV can be transmitted by contaminated needles or other objects that penetrate the skin. AIDS is now very much a disease of women. Large numbers are being infected from heterosexual and bisexual partners. Between one and 10 years after infection 80% of

people develop AIDS, or a widespread lymph node problem, or brain involvement. Fifty per cent will develop the full AIDS pattern, with such severe loss of immunity that they become susceptible to a wide range of infections and some cancers. Most of these can be controlled for a time, but the established condition is virtually always fatal.

### The AIDS-related complex

This is a syndrome that affects a considerable proportion of HIV-positive people. The most striking feature is enlargement of the lymph nodes, occurring on both sides of the body and in three or more sites, indicating that the enlargement is not due to local infection in the area drained by a particular group of nodes. There is also enlargement of the liver and the spleen and a variety of different skin rashes. These rashes are all of types commonly seen in other conditions and are due to a reduction in resistance to common infections. Thus, patients with ARC may develop multiple small boils or pimples, impetigo, shingles (from earlier acquired chicken-pox virus) and fungus infections such as 'ringworm' (*tinea*) or thrush.

These are the symptoms of the minor form of ARC and clinical experience suggests that such people are unlikely to develop the full AIDS picture for some years. There is, however, a more severe form in which the signs described are complicated by considerable loss of weight, persistent diarrhoea, fever and perhaps a heavy thrush infection of the mouth and genitals. The indications are that such people are more likely to progress more quickly to AIDS.

### Fully developed AIDS

AIDS develops in about 54% of HIV-positive people within 10

years of infection and develops eventually in virtually all. Whether or not AIDS develops at any point depends on how badly the immune system is damaged. Any other factors which affect the efficiency of the immune system are important. Even heavy alcohol consumption or pregnancy may tip the balance in favour of the full-blown immune deficiency syndrome. Also, a person who deliberately and repeatedly exposes herself to further infection with HIV is likely to have trouble at an earlier stage than one who does not.

In fully developed AIDS, immunity has, for practical purposes, been lost, and infecting organisms, both those which commonly cause disease and those which would not normally be able to do so, can gain a foothold in the body and proceed, relatively unchecked, to cause massive infection. For most of the common infecting agents, antibiotics and chemotherapeutic drugs are available and these are, in general, effective. When such infections occur in people with AIDS, they are in no way different, except perhaps in severity, from those in other people and they are treated in exactly the same way.

But treatment is usually less effective for what are known as the 'opportunistic' organisms. These are viruses, bacteria, fungi and protozoa (single-celled animal parasites, sometimes amoebic) which are able to get a hold in the body only if not opposed by a normal immune system. The pattern of opportunistic infection in AIDS is well known and the frequency of the various infections established. Many different effects occur and only some of these can be described here.

### *Cytomegalovirus* infection

The cytomegalovirus (CMV) is a herpes virus which does not

normally cause any problems. In AIDS it is the commonest opportunistic infection. It causes:

- extensive skin rashes
- a form of pneumonia which, in severe cases, can be fatal
- inflammation of the liver with disturbance of liver function and possibly jaundice
- fever
- night sweating
- internal damage to the eyes involving the retinas so that permanent visual loss may result
- inflammation of the brain (*encephalitis*) which may cause permanent damage to brain function

Cytomegalovirus is hard to treat but the drug gancyclovir is of some value. It is, unfortunately, toxic.

### Candidiasis

The next most common infection in AIDS, affecting about half of all patients, is thrush (*candidiasis*). This is, of course, an everyday infection in people with normal immune systems, especially women, in whom vaginal thrush is very common. But the immune system always prevents the infection from getting completely out of hand and it is rare for thrush to spread widely and to involve the deeply internal parts of the body.

In AIDS the situation is very different. Freed from immunological control, the fungus spreads like wild-fire, commonly extending down from the mouth into the gullet (*oesophagus*) where ulceration occurs, causing severe difficulty and pain on swallowing. The whole of the genital and anal area may be covered with the white fungus and the inside of the mouth thickly coated. Occasionally, the yeast gets into the bloodstream and is carried to any part of the body to set up a focus of infection. Most commonly involved are the eyes, the kidneys and the skin.

There is a reasonably effective range of drugs for candidiasis, and the skin involvement, especially, will respond fairly well to drugs such as Canesten (clotrimazole), Miconazole, Nystatin, amphotericin B and Ketoconazole.

### *Pneumocystis carinii* pneumonia

Pneumocystis is a single-celled parasite which hardly ever causes trouble in people with normal immune systems. But in those who are immunocompromised, the organism frequently produces a dangerous infection. In AIDS patients the trouble starts with a persistent, annoying, dry cough and breathlessness on quite minor effort. Characteristically, a formerly fit person becomes breathless even when at rest. The disease process is having a serious effect in that it is preventing the normal amount of oxygen from getting through from the atmosphere to the blood. Tests of the amount of oxygen in the blood will show that this is unusually low and this is why people with this condition are often breathless and sometimes show a bluish colour in the skin (*cyanosis*).

In the lungs, a thick frothy liquid forms in the air sacs and this prevents the air from reaching the thin-walled blood vessels through which it should pass to get into the blood. The condition is dangerous because very rapid deterioration can occur if it is not diagnosed quickly and treated, and the outcome is sometimes fatal. Specific treatment is available but early diagnosis is vital.

**Herpes simplex**
Herpes in the immune deficiency state is an extension of the relatively minor inconvenience of genital herpes or cold sores around the mouth. The uncontrolled spread of herpes in AIDS is a very painful and distressing effect of the compromised immune system. It is, essentially, an exaggeration of the herpes infection well known to many, featuring painful, tense, opalescent blisters around the mouth or nose, or spreading around the skin of the vulva, anus and buttocks. In AIDS, the effects are not confined to these sites but spread inward, both locally and remotely, to involve the inside of the mouth, the gullet and even the windpipe and air passages of the respiratory tract. The blisters also spread into the rectum and the urinary system causing severe pain, difficulty in urination or defaecation and alteration in sensation around the buttocks.

Remote spread is even more serious as this often leads to involvement of the brain, causing inflammation of the brain (*herpes encephalitis*) and inflammation of the brain linings (*herpes meningitis*). These are, of course, grave complications. The most successful drug, to date, against herpes simplex is Zovirax (acyclovir).

*Toxoplasma gondii* **infection**
Human infection with this single-celled parasite is widespread. Most people harbour some of the organisms, harmlessly. Many, however, have small foci of the infection in the eyes and these occasionally flare up and sometimes cause

damage to vision. The case is much more serious in the immunocompromised and, in AIDS, the chief danger is to the brain. About 10% of AIDS victims are affected in this way causing small and widespread foci or a large abscess-like mass. If the patient survives, there is usually a slowly progressive dementia that often becomes seriously disabling. *T. gondii* can also cause pneumonia and, like cytomegalovirus, commonly affects the vision.

Treatment is difficult, for the organism is very resistant and the best currently available drugs are not very effective. So prevention of new infection is very important in immunocompromised people. Toxoplasmosis is commonly acquired from undercooked meat, so all sorts of meat, game and fish should be thoroughly cooked. Another important source of infection is domestic cats, who commonly acquire the toxoplasma. Infected cats excrete the cystic collections of *T. gondii* in their droppings and these are highly infectious. Immunocompromised people should not keep cats and should keep away from cat boxes or soil used by cats.

### Kaposi's sarcoma

This is a multiple tumour of blood vessels, primarily affecting the skin, usually on the lower limbs and growing very slowly. Kaposi's sarcoma affects about a quarter of the men with AIDS. It is relatively rare in women. The visible spots are small, circular and pinkish or reddish, usually situated on the legs and buttocks. Sometimes the spots are more raised and appear as nodules or plaques of a bluish-purple to dark brown colour. They vary in size from a few millimetres to one centimetre across and vary in number from one to hundreds.

Kaposi's sarcoma is often found, at an early stage, to have involved the insides of the bowels, the mouth, the lungs, the lymph nodes or, indeed, almost any organ of the body. Some of these spots seem quiescent, but some may become locally destructive, ulcerating through the skin into the deeper tissues and even sometimes involving the underlying bone.

A fair proportion of people with AIDS have shown no other signs of immune deficiency. But the discovery of Kaposi's sarcoma in a young person with opportunistic infections is an alarming indication of the severity of the immune deficiency and few such patients survive longer than two years, once the diagnosis is confirmed.

### Outlook

Although all the manifestations of AIDS can be treated, there is still no effective treatment for the HIV infection itself, nor any effective vaccine. Although a very small proportion of HIV-positive people do not appear to develop AIDS, almost all do, sooner or later. Once the condition is fully established, the outlook is virtually hopeless. See also SEXUALLY TRANSMITTED DISEASES.

## Alphafetoprotein

This is a protein formed in the liver and intestine of every fetus and present in fetal blood. Small quantities of alphafetoprotein are passed into the fluid in the UTERUS (*amniotic fluid*) and are swallowed by the fetus. Some of it thus gets into the mother's blood, by way of the placenta. The levels of alphafetoprotein rise as the pregnancy advances and can be detected in the mother's blood from the third month onward. If the levels are greatly raised this may indicate that the fetus has spina bifida or a serious brain disorder (*anencephaly*) and further investigation becomes urgent. ULTRASOUND SCANNING and possibly AMNIOCENTESIS must be done.

Levels may also be raised in certain fetal kidney and bowel conditions, in multiple pregnancy, and in threatened or actual ABORTION. The levels may, wrongly, seem abnormally high if there has been a mistake in the pregnancy dates.

Raised alphafetoprotein levels are also found in most people with cancer of the liver or testicle and in some with cancer of the bowel.

## Amenorrhoea

Absence of menstruation. This is normal before puberty and after the menopause. During the reproductive years, the commonest cause is pregnancy and lactation (milk secretion), but it can be caused by a number of hormonal and other disorders, by excessive athletic activity or by ANOREXIA NERVOSA. See also PERIOD PROBLEMS.

## Amniocentesis

This is a way of finding out whether a fetus has a genetic or other disorder. The test is usually done between the 16th and 20th weeks of pregnancy. Under local anaesthesia and ultrasonic viewing, a needle is passed carefully through the wall of the abdomen and the wall of the UTERUS into the amniotic fluid in which the fetus is floating. A sample of fluid is then withdrawn. Because this fluid contains cells shed from the skin of the fetus and various substances secreted by the fetus, samples obtained contain DNA and can be of the greatest importance for diagnosis.

Alphafetoprotein levels in the amniotic fluid can give reliable information on the likelihood of congenital defects in the spinal cord and column (*spina bifida*) and absence of part of the fetal brain (*anencephaly*). Levels in the mother's blood are also measured routinely. Cells from the amniotic fluid can be grown in tissue cultures so that the chromosomes can be checked after three or four weeks. In this way, Down's syndrome and a great range of other genetic diseases, can be detected before birth. It is possible to diagnose cystic fibrosis, factor VIII and factor IX types of haemophilia, some forms of muscular dystrophy, thalassaemia, sickle cell anaemia, antitrypsin deficiency and phenylketonuria. Later in pregnancy amniocentesis provides information directly about the likelihood of a number of conditions, such as rhesus factor disease and the respiratory distress syndrome.

Amniocentesis does carry a small risk to the fetus and is not done without good reason. It may cause abortion if done early. It may damage the afterbirth (*placenta*) or the fetus and may cause bleeding into the amniotic fluid. The risk of fetal death from amniocentesis is less than 1%. Sexing of the future child is not a justification for the procedure, however anxious the future parents may be to know.

Such early methods of detection of serious or potentially serious major disorders give parents the option of an early termination of the pregnancy. They also sometimes provide the opportunity for early treatment of the disorder while the fetus remains in the uterus.

## Anaemia

A reduction in the amount of the oxygen-carrying iron and protein material, haemoglobin, in the red blood cells. Because a good supply of oxygen is so vital, anaemia has widespread effects, causing weakness, fatigue, tiredness and breathlessness on minor effort. The skin may appear pale and there is lowered resistance to infection.

There are several different kinds of anaemia including simple iron deficiency anaemia, haemolytic anaemia, pernicious anaemia and aplastic anaemia. In women, by far the commonest cause is excessive menstrual loss of blood coupled with an inadequate iron intake. Anaemia may also occur because of the extra nutritional demands of pregnancy. Treatment is based on the cause and usually involves no more than supplementary iron.

## Anger

Anger is a common emotion and a major cause of unhappiness. If the ultimate aim of the medical profession is to relieve distress and promote human happiness, the neglect of the study of anger is inexplicable. Anger has enormous individual and social implications. Marriages are turned to misery, wives are battered. Violence in the home is, almost always, a manifestation of anger.

Anger does not necessarily lead to physical aggression against others. It may be manifested by verbal abuse, by violent action against the self, dangerous behaviour often in a car, repression and building up of resentment, cutting off from any form of communication, running away, withdrawing into apathy, overeating.

# ANGER

Anger starts with the perception of a wrong and is concerned with attempts to put it right. The perception is, of course, a very individual one and may be at odds with other people's perception of the same situation. Anger limits clear thinking and leads to impulsive action, which is often regretted. It may give an illusory sense of being in control of a situation and lead to action which makes things worse.

People prone to anger are often people literally looking for trouble. They are very much concerned with their perception of other people's attitudes to them, take everything personally, have an often quite unrealistic idea of what the world ought to be like and feel themselves entitled to try to change it. Many such people anticipate or assume that encounters will be hostile, attributing aggressive attitudes to others. They enjoy working out punishments for others and justifying themselves.

It is important to appreciate that it is not the perceived event or apparent external stimulus that causes the anger, but the nature of the perception itself – the way people interpret what is happening to them. The 'internal speech' of the anger-prone is full of aggressive dialogue, self-justifying value judgements and imagined successful put-downs.

Predictably, few angry people are willing to recognize that they have a problem and submit to treatment. But when anger has led to behaviour that even the aggressor recognizes as socially unacceptable, treatment is sometimes welcomed. The most effective form of treatment is a kind of behaviour therapy that makes much use of acted role-playing techniques. First the subject is made to look critically at anger, to understand its functions and effects, to distinguish between the emotion of anger and its outward effects and to recognize the kind of behaviour patterns that lead to escalation. The next stage involves learning how to analyse thoughts and feelings, recognize common logical fallacies, deal with personal relationships and achieve more effective communication. The final stage is to discover, first by role-play and then in real life, how effectively these lessons have been learnt.

## Anorexia nervosa

'Anorexia' simply means 'loss of appetite' something experienced by most people from time to time. But anorexia nervosa is a serious disorder of perception that causes the sufferer, almost always a young woman, to believe that she is too fat, when, in fact, she is actually very thin. The result, inevitably, is severe emaciation. Anorexia nervosa is common in models, actresses, dancers and others who are much concerned with the appearance of their bodies. In a minority of cases it is a symptom of a serious underlying psychiatric disorder such as severe depression or schizophrenia.

The cause of anorexia is still a matter of debate. Many anorexics come from close-knit families and have a particularly intimate relationship with one parent. They are often obsessional in their habits. They are conformists and usually anxious to please. Some seem unwilling to grow up and appear to be trying to retain their childhood shape. Others seem to have a genuine fatness phobia with fear of eating fats or carbohydrates. Social factors probably contribute, especially the common and entirely arbitrary identification of slimness with sexual attractiveness. Such influences may powerfully affect girls who are deeply concerned with how they are regarded by others.

Medically, the effects of anorexia nervosa, often hidden by the sufferer in the early stages, are obvious. The signs of starvation are unfortunately only too clear. When calorie intake is less than energy expenditure and the needs of structural replacement, first the fat stores are used up and then the muscles are used for fuel. In anorexia there is extreme thinness with loss of a third or more of the body weight. There is, inevitably, severe tiredness and weakness and often the effects of vitamin deficiency. The skin becomes dry and the hair falls out. Early in the process there is, in almost all cases, absence of menstruation. Death from starvation, or suicide, is common.

Anorexia nervosa demands skilled treatment in hospital under the care of those experienced in the condition. Personality problems and the persistence of the disorder can make treatment difficult. Management depends on psychotherapy and insistence on re-feeding. Patients will usually make every effort to circumvent treatment, holding food in their mouths until it can be disposed of. Strict control is essential. Unless a watch is kept, food will be hidden or secretly thrown away. Often a system of rewards may be effective, in which privileges, such as visits or leave passes, are awarded for weight gained.

Antidepressant drugs are often helpful in the early stages. Even after normal weight has been regained, young women who have had anorexia nervosa may need to remain under psychiatric care for months or years. Relapses are common and, tragically, up to 10% later die from suicide or starvation.

## Anovulation

Failure of the ovaries to produce normal eggs so that conception is impossible. This may result from hormonal or other disease or from natural states such as pregnancy and lactation (milk production). Women taking combined oral contraceptives do not ovulate while taking the pills. See also INFERTILITY.

## Anxiety

Anxiety is a natural response to threat or danger, whether real or imagined. When people are anxious their bodies produce certain hormones, which, while helping to cope with the danger, also cause some very unpleasant symptoms.

The persistently worried state of mind involves being constantly 'keyed up'. This causes:

- an exaggerated startle response
- lack of concentration
- irritability
- insomnia
- a tendency for the mind to 'go blank'

Closely related to these mental effects are the corresponding physical manifestations. These are many, and include:

- a rapid pulse
- muscle tension
- tooth-grinding (*bruxism*)
- restlessness
- easy fatiguability
- breathlessness

- tremulousness
- palpitations
- a feeling of tightness in the chest
- sweating
- clammy hands
- dry mouth
- nausea
- diarrhoea
- flushing
- frequency of urination
- a 'lump in the throat'

There is narrowing of attention and reduced mental efficiency with disorganisation and poor performance. Doctors are still arguing whether these symptoms are the effect of the state of mind or are the cause of it.

Severe anxiety that occurs without any obvious cause is abnormal, disabling and very common. Terms describing such states quickly become derogatory and some doctors, for reasons of sympathy, keep changing them. Anxiety states or anxiety neuroses have become *free-floating* anxiety. Hypochondriasis has become a *psychosomatic disorder*. And phobias have become *situational anxiety*.

Anxiety often seems deeply rooted in the personality. Many anxious people are convinced that their symptoms are due to organic disease. The physical symptoms of anxiety help to promote the belief that there is heart disease, cancer or AIDS. These unfortunate people often undergo repeated and fruitless medical investigation. Some become psychologically dependent on doctors who are kind to them and on tranquillizing drugs. They do not always get effective treatment.

Many of the symptoms of anxiety can be relieved. Beta blockers and antihistamine drugs are often very effective. The benzodiazepine drugs like Valium and Librium were once widely used, but their disadvantages – dependency and addiction – are now apparent and they are being replaced by newer 'anxiolytic' drugs, for which better things are claimed. Tricyclic and monoamine oxidase inhibiting antidepressant drugs have some part to play in the treatment of anxiety.

Anxiety may also be a symptom of various other conditions including thyroid overactivity (see THYROID GLAND DISORDERS), menopausal hormonal disturbances, drug withdrawal, schizophrenia, depressive illness, post-concussional syndrome and dementia. Long-term anxiety, however, is unlikely to be due to organic disorder.

# B

## Backache

Lumbago, or low back pain, is one of the commonest and most persistent of symptoms. It is especially common in pregnancy and following childbirth. The idea that backache is caused by a turned-back (*retroverted*) uterus is no longer believed. Most cases are due to faulty posture and to the maintenance, after pregnancy, of the forward bend in the lower spine (*lordosis*), which is an inevitable feature of late pregnancy. Cases caused in this way will usually clear up soon after delivery, especially if attention is given to the posture.

It is a mistake, however to assume that backache is necessarily associated with pregnancy. Many cases occur at other times. The symptom becomes more frequent with age, and about half of all those over sixty suffer frequently from it. In most of these cases it is also due to a defective, slouching posture associated with poor development in the large group of muscles surrounding the spine (*paravertebral muscles*). Backache caused in this way can usually be relieved by exercises to strengthen the muscles and by the adoption of a proper, upright posture, both in standing and in sitting. Often, this type of backache is brought on, or made worse, by obesity or by unaccustomed or injudicious work or weight-bearing.

The fibrous connective tissue of the back muscles, ligaments and tendons is often the site of pain and this may follow unusual or strenuous exercise, especially in sport in the untrained. Lumbar pain can also be related to mental stress, virus infections, sleep disorders and anxiety.

The most common serious form of back pain is caused by what is popularly described as 'slipped disc'. This is an inaccurate term as the discs between the bodies of the vertebrae of the spine are very securely attached to the bone and cannot slip. Even the official medical term – prolapsed intervertebral disc – is not quite right. It is not the disc that is displaced, but a variable quantity of the soft, pulpy central material (*nucleus pulposus*) which is forced by longitudinal pressure through a localized defect in the outer fibrous ring of the disc and squashed backwards to press on the spinal nerves. Pressure on these nerves causes, not only severe backache, but also pain which radiates down the course of the nerve – through the buttock, back of the thigh and down as far as the foot. These nerves are bundled together to form the main nerve trunk supplying the leg (*sciatic nerve*) and pressure on them causes not only severe backache but sciatica. Severe backache and stiffness associated with involvement of the sciatic nerve – pain, numbness or loss of function – indicate a prolapsed disc and call for proper medical or surgical treatment.

There are many other causes of backache, but these are much less common. They include:

- a tear of a muscle or ligament
- an actual fracture of one of the facets or processes of a vertebra
- wearing away of the joint surfaces (*chronic osteoarthritis*)
- inflammation of the spine (*ankylosing spondylitis*)
- minor abnormalities of the lower part of the spine present from birth (congenital bone defects)
- a slipping forward of the lowest lumbar vertebra on the top of the sacrum (*spondylolisthesis*)

- bone tuberculosis
- bone marrow cancer (*myeloma*) or secondary cancer which has spread to the bone

Most attacks of acute low back pain settle in a few days, but it is important to try to determine and avoid the cause as, otherwise, recurrence is likely. This may lead to a permanent (*chronic*) situation. In severe and persistent cases it is essential to seek medical advice so that a correct diagnosis can be reached and appropriate treatment given. Backache is a *symptom* – an indication of something else, not a disease in its own right.

Osteopaths believe that many backaches are caused by actual displacement of one vertebra relative to another and that they can be relieved by identifying the site of the dislocation and applying pressure to reduce it. Certainly, many people have been relieved of their backache by osteopathic treatment, but most doctors are sceptical of the claimed cause. A good osteopath will probably know more about backache than most doctors, but there is always the worry that treatment will be undertaken without an accurate diagnosis. This can be dangerous, if only by delaying access to proper management.

## Bartholin's glands

Between the back part of the vaginal opening and the LABIA minora on either side, lie the openings of the two reddish-yellow Bartholin's glands, each about half an inch long and lying under the labia majora. Sexual excitement causes these glands to secrete a crystal-clear mucin that lubricates the vaginal opening and is a great help during intercourse. These glands sometimes become infected and may form painful abscesses that have to be opened surgically.

The glands are named after the Danish anatomist, Caspar Bartholin (1655–1738), who first described their function in 1679.

## Bisexuality

The inclination for sexual intercourse with either men or women. Bisexual behaviour is common, but genuine neutrality in the choice of sex objects is very rare. Bisexual behaviour occurs in both sexes and among those with heterosexual as well as homosexual preference. Often it seems to be a matter of force of circumstance in closed communities such as boarding schools, prisons and so on. Prostitutes often prefer a lesbian relationship for emotional outlet even if they are heterosexually active in their private lives.

Kinsey used a realistic scale of 0-6 for assessing the range of sexuality from exclusively heterosexual to exclusively homosexual. A study of the placement of his subjects on this scale suggests that about 20% of women and 30% of men were capable of, or had engaged in, bisexual activity. Sometimes bisexual behaviour is a consequence of an apparently ungovernable appetite for orgasm. In these cases it seems likely that the true psychosexual orientation is irrelevant.

## Bladder

See URINARY PROBLEMS.

## Blushing

Blushing is a transient reddening of the face, ears and neck, often spreading to the upper part of the chest, but rarely, if ever, to more remote parts of the body. The skin contains an extensive network of small arteries with smooth muscle fibres in their walls. Normally, these muscles are in a state of partial contraction. Extreme contraction causes the arteries to close down so that less blood flows through the skin and it becomes pale. Full relaxation of these muscles causes widening of the blood vessels and a larger quantity of blood than normal passes through the skin causing flushing, or blushing.

These tiny artery muscles are controlled by nerves of the non-voluntary (*autonomic*) nervous system and this, in turn, is affected by various influences, including the emotions. Any strong tendency to blush, as in adolescence, may thus be due both to emotional instability and to undue sensitivity of the autonomic system. Adolescent blushing commonly ceases to be a problem with maturity and growing social confidence.

Widening of blood vessels is a feature of sexual excitement, especially in women, and a widespread mottled flush commonly occurs during sexual intercourse. The hot flushes of the menopause are also caused by blood vessels widening. In this case, the stimulus to the autonomic system is a deficiency of the female sex hormone, oestrogen.

Blushing can become a permanent problem. The disease acne rosacea (not to be confused with common acne) is a state of permanent widening of the blood vessels of the skin of the cheeks and nose. There are effective treatments for this condition.

## Body development
There is really not a great deal of physical difference between

little girls and little boys. The differences start to appear at puberty. This is the period, some time between 10 and 14, when a girl's sexual organs enlarge and become capable of use and her body gradually acquires the appearance of a woman. The significance of sexuality begins to become apparent, along with the realization that she has become capable of having babies. Puberty usually takes three or four years. It starts at different ages in different girls and proceed at different speeds. Maybe you were surprised to note how some of your friends were at very different stages of development. These differences were transitional, however, and eventually the 'late developers' caught up.

The last event in female puberty is the beginning of the periods. On average, this occurs about age 13, but the periods can start as early as nine or as late as 16. The age of onset has been getting gradually lower in the Western world for at least 100 years, dropping by about a month in every 10 years. This change has now stabilized and was probably due to improving nutrition.

Puberty is caused by oestrogen hormones from the ovaries. These are produced in small quantities throughout childhood, but really get going when the pituitary gland suddenly prompts the ovaries into high-level oestrogen production. They do this by secreting hormones called gonadotrophins – a complicated word that simply means 'making the sex glands grow'. Oestrogens are the female sex hormones and are responsible for the development of female characteristics.

The changes brought about by oestrogens usually occur in

a fairly standard order. They are:

- breast budding
- growth of pubic hair
- growth of underarm hair
- production of underarm sweat
- increased breast development and size equalization
- development and maturation of the ovaries
- widening of the pelvis
- deposition of fat on hips, thighs, buttocks and breasts
- a spurt in body growth
- muscular development
- a tendency to acne
- egg (*ovum*) production by the ovaries (*ovulation*)
- the first menstrual period
- regular menstrual periods

Sometimes the first few menstrual periods occur before ovulation starts. Adolescence is the time between the start of puberty and point of full adult physical development. Most girls will have reached some 80% of the final adult height at the time of puberty, but during puberty and early adolescence a considerable growth spurt will probably have occurred. At the same time there is a considerable increase in the weight of fat and muscle. By the age of 18 it is likely that as much as 20% of the total weight will be in fat. This is a considerably higher proportion of total weight than in the average young man of the same age. This has nothing to do with obesity. Fat deposits in young women are important secondary sexual characteristics and are largely responsible for the natural difference in body shape between women and men.

Just occasionally puberty goes wrong. Puberty coming too early (*precocious puberty*) usually does little physical harm, but sometimes the growing zones of the long bones (*epiphyses*) will also shut down early, leaving you a bit on the short side. It is, however, sometimes psychologically disturbing. Unduly delayed puberty may result from under-development of the sexual organs. So a very late puberty should always be medically investigated. Treatment may be needed if the periods have not started by the age of 18.

It is quite common for the early periods to be very heavy, but this usually rights itself. Sometimes a combined oral contraceptive pill may be needed for two or three cycles, to sort this out.

Apart from the sexual differences in body size, shape and weight, there are some very fundamental structural differences between the bodies of women and those of men. The most obvious of these are in the genitalia. This term usually refers to the external genitalia – the LABIA majora and minora and the CLITORIS, but, strictly speaking, the genitalia also include all the organs of reproduction – the VAGINA, UTERUS, FALLOPIAN TUBES and OVARIES.

## Body odour

An unpleasant and usually socially unacceptable smell most commonly caused by the action of bacteria on the sweat produced by the apocrine sweat glands of the armpits and the groin areas and on moist skin debris generally. The remedy for this form of body odour is daily washing and, if necessary, the use of a sweat-retarding deodorant (see DEODORANTS).

Minor body odour can also arise from the vulva, if there is persistent infection of the VAGINA with the organism *Gardnerella vaginalis*. This produces a characteristic fishy smell, especially when in contact with mild alkalis, as in soap. A course of Flagyl (metronidazole) will soon put this right.

Some volatile substances taken by mouth are excreted in the sweat in sufficient quantity to make their presence felt to others. These include alcohol, garlic and tobacco products.

## Breast

Your breasts are glandular organs with two main functions – to attract men and to secrete milk. Medically, they are correctly described as mammary glands. Both sexes have rudimentary breasts at birth and in the male, the breast remains rudimentary. At puberty, however, female sex hormones cause breasts to grow, NIPPLES to enlarge and fat to be deposited under the breast skin. The nipple occurs at the tip of each breast and is surrounded by a coloured area, about 3.75 cm in diameter called the areola. This enlarges and darkens in colour, and full development of the breast occurs, during pregnancy.

Each of your breasts consists of a round mass of glandular tissue divided into 15 to 20 lobes. Each lobe has a milk duct leading to an opening on the nipple. The size of your breasts is determined more by the amount of fat than by the amount of glandular tissue. Strands of protein called connective tissue form a kind of skeleton for the breast and these strands are connected to the flat pectoral muscles under the breast.

## Breast abscess

Breast inflammation (*mastitis*) is common during breastfeeding because the nipples often suffer injury and abrasion. Germs pass into the breast by way of these abrasions and set up an infection. There is painful swelling in the affected breast, redness, tenderness, tension and often inability to pass milk. Soon the breast becomes extremely swollen, there is fever and general upset and the lymph nodes in the armpit swell and become tender. General breast tenderness and tension are normal features of the first few days of lactation, but any local tenderness, redness or pain must be reported at once.

Mastitis that is not properly treated with antibiotics may rapidly progress to abscess, but this may occur even if antibiotics are given. One or more areas of softening and local tissue destruction occur and collections of pus form. At this stage a minor surgical operation is necessary to open abscesses and release the pus. Milk production must be stopped with hormones.

## Breast augmentation

Strong cultural pressures are still imposed on women to conform to current notions of the optimum size and shape of the breast. The same pressures can induce dissatisfaction. Breasts may displease because they are too small, too pendulous, too large, too heavy or, perhaps most important, lacking in symmetry. Ideally, the bulk of the breasts should be in proportion to the other body dimensions and to the general quality of the build. And there are other features, such as fullness, roundness, good nipple positioning and symmetry, which are more or less universally accepted as desirable.

Cosmetic surgery will be unsatisfactory if it achieves only an alteration in the outline of the breasts but does not preserve the normal consistency and 'feel'. The breast has much of the characteristics of a fluid-filled bag. Its shape and position are greatly affected by gravity, so it will alter markedly with changes in the position of the body and on raising the arms. It also changes with contraction of the underlying pectoral muscles and on deep breathing. The shape of your breasts when you are lying on your back, is quite different from when you are on hands and knees. The ability of the breasts to alter in this way must be preserved or the effect will be very unnatural.

The position of the darker circle surrounding the nipple (*areola*) and of the nipple itself must be acceptable and surgery should not, if possible, interfere with the sensitivity of this part to touch. The nipple should be of adequate size and projection and the ability to breast feed should, if possible, be retained. Turned in (inverted) nipples can be turned outward fairly easily. Breast enlargement (*augmentation mammoplasty*) can usually be done while satisfying all these criteria; it is much less easy to reduce breasts without diminishing sensation and interfering with lactation.

Small, or almost absent, breasts often induce a sense of sexual inferiority. The desire for the boyish, flat-chested look has, generally, yielded to an acknowledgement of the secondary sexual characteristics, and there is considerable demand for surgery to increase the size of the breast. A woman's image of her own body, and even her sense of her own worth, may be damaged by what she perceives as breast inadequacies. The longing of these women for fuller breasts can only be satisfied by artificial enlargement. After successful surgical treatment, nearly all women are able to forget that something has been inserted under the skin and can incorporate the new shape into their own body image and identity.

It is important to appreciate that not all women with small breasts are suitable for augmentation. Difficulties may be encountered if breasts have formerly been of satisfactory size but have, as a result of loss of fat, become flat and drooping. Breasts of this kind should not be treated by simple implant augmentation, as the implant will just sag down like a cannon ball in a sack. A different operation altogether is required, in which redundant skin is removed. This is called *mastopexy*. The general rule is that if, when you are sitting upright, your nipples lie at a level below the crease at which the breast joins your chest, simple augmentation should not be done, unless combined with a mastopexy.

### How is augmentation done?

It would be a serious mistake just to slip the implant under the skin. This would be asking for trouble. The implant would simply ulcerate through to the outside. Implants must be buried as deeply as possible, certainly behind the fat and breast tissue and, according to some surgeons, preferably even behind the flat pectoral muscles which lie deep to the breast. The operation may be done either under local or general anaesthesia and the incision is almost always made on the under-side of the breast just a little in front of the crease. The incision is about one and a half inches long. The surgeon then carefully separates the tissues so as to form a pocket behind the breast. This pocket is then enlarged with the gloved finger until it can comfortably accommodate the implant. Any bleeding is firmly checked, for *haematoma* (collection of blood in a large clot) must be avoided. The implant is then pushed into the pocket and the incision closed with a few stitches. If an inflatable implant is used, the incision may be smaller.

Silicone rubber has long been regarded as an outstanding material for surgical implants and has been successfully used, for all sorts of supporting and structural purposes, in many parts of the body. It is used as a standard material for the treatment of retinal detachment and has proved itself stable and generally safe. After unhappy experience with all sorts of implant materials for breasts, the major advance in augmentation mammoplasty seemed to have finally arrived in 1963. This advance was the development of an implant consisting of a silicone rubber capsule loosely filled with a soft silicone jelly. This method proved more satisfactory than any other and has been widely used. Millions of women have had the operation using this kind of implant. Up to as late as 1990, some 100,000 American women were having silicone implants each year for cosmetic reasons.

In the early 1980s, however, disquieting reports had begun to appear about a possible association between silicone implants and three diseases of the autoimmune group. These were rheumatoid arthritis, systemic lupus erythematosus – a condition that damages the skin, joints and various internal organs – and scleroderma – a disfiguring hardening of the skin that can also affect the organs. In 1988 the American *Food and Drugs Administration* (FDA), which had become responsible for the safety of medical devices in 1976, began to ask manufacturers of breast implants to provide them with data about their safety. In 1991 a US Federal Court found that a major manufacturer had concealed evidence concerning the link between ruptured silicone implants and these diseases. And on 6th January 1992 the FDA asked doctors to stop silicone gel implants while the evidence was reviewed. Silicone implants containing saline were not affected by the ruling.

Arguments continued for some time, but it gradually became clear that liquid silicone leaking from implants was exciting a reaction in the body from the immune system. Later research showed that some women with implants were producing antinuclear antibodies – the type associated with autoimmune disease and which attack the body's own tissues. The proportion of women affected in this way was small. A paper in *The Lancet* of 28th November, 1992 reported that about 88 cases of autoimmune-type disease associated with breast augmentation had been reported. The number of women who have had implants runs into millions. The main danger seems to be when implants rupture and release the gel into the tissues. Unfortunately, the silicone capsule itself causes local reactions leading to hardening of tissue and doctors have been advising deliberate breaking up of this hardened tissue (see below).

These results put women who have had silicone gel implants into a very difficult position and tens of thousands have made the heartbreaking decision to have their implants removed.

### Other complications of augmentation
Haematoma is an early complication and causes one or both breasts to continue to swell painfully. It would be uncommon

to have this happen on both sides, but anything is possible. Haematomas must be removed without delay as they may to lead to abscess formation and later scar formation with contractures and unsatisfactory breast shape. Even if they do not become infected, scarring is likely. So if a haematoma develops, the patient has to go back to theatre for drainage and control of further bleeding.

About one woman in six notices that after the operation the sensitivity of the nipples is changed. Sometimes the sensation is reduced, but often there is a tingling or tickling sensation which may persist for several months. Occasionally there is permanent total loss of sensation. This is quite distressing to some women. Incidentally, the danger of loss of nipple sensation is much greater following breast reduction than following augmentation.

The main long-term complication of augmentation mammoplasty is the development of a hard fibrous capsule around the implant, leading to an unnatural and undesirable feel in the breast and even some distortion of its shape. This is usually noticed within about six months of the operation, but may occur even years afterwards. The complication is very common – about one woman in four experiences it – and your surgeon may try to prevent this from happening by giving you an injection of steroids into the breasts at the time of the implant and by instructing you in the art of daily breast massage. If, in spite of these measures, the fibrosis does occur, your surgeon may recommend forcible break-up of the fibrous capsule, by powerful external squeezing – a rather bruising ordeal – or even the surgical removal and replacement of the implant. In view of the danger of leakage, such a measure is not recommended in the case of silicone gel implants.

These complications don't usually seem to detract much from the satisfaction most women derive from augmentation. But just one final word of warning. If you are in the market for breast enhancement, do be sure that it is you who wants it done, not someone else. The basic impulse really must come from you.

### Breast cancer

This is the commonest form of cancer in women and a very common disease, affecting about one woman in 14 in Britain. It is the leading cause of death among women between 40 and 55 years of age in the USA. In Japan, by contrast, the incidence is only about one fifth that in the USA. The medical literature on the subject is enormous and many hundreds, if not thousands of trials of all kinds, connected with the disease, have been done. As a result statistics on breast cancer are very complicated and sometimes contradictory. It is difficult to get entirely reliable figures and any quoted here should be taken as only approximate.

Breast cancer is rare before the age of 30 and the incidence rises rapidly during the 40s. After the menopause, the incidence continues to rise with age, but less rapidly. About one third of cases occur under the age of 50, one third between 50 and 64 and one third in women over 64. The risk of breast cancer is doubled if the mother had it, and is increased about three times in those who have already had it in one breast. Again, figures are uncertain and vary with the individual.

Other less important risk factors are believed to be:

- having no children
- starting menstruation early
- exposure to radiation
- being in a high socioeconomic group
- eating a high-fat diet
- taking large doses of oestrogens
- taking oral contraceptives
- tallness
- alcohol intake
- having had cancer of the ovaries or of the lining of the UTERUS.

The risk is believed to be doubled in women who habitually drink three units of alcohol a day. Women with many children and those who have had their ovaries removed (*oophorectomy*) are less likely, than average, to get breast cancer.

Breast cancers are insidious and hardly ever cause pain. There may, sometimes, be a vague discomfort, but, commonly, the only sign is the finding of a slowly growing lump. There are, however, other possible signs and these should be known and looked for. They are:

- distortion of the normal breast contour by skin dimpling
- indrawing, or alteration in direction, of the nipple
- bleeding from the nipple
- distortion of the area around the nipple (*areola*)
- orange-skin texture appearance (*peau d'orange*) of the breast skin
- alteration in the position or hang of the breast compared to the other side

- rubbery, firm, easily felt glands (lymph nodes) in the armpit

Breast cancer can spread directly, or by passing along lymph channels, to and through the lymph nodes or even by way of the bloodstream. Remote spread is usually to the lungs, bones and liver. Minimal breast cancers are those confined to the milk ducts and lobes of the breast. They remain in the original location (*in situ*) for a long time before becoming invasive and spreading outside the breast and are easily curable if detected. They nearly always occur in pre-menopausal women. Unfortunately they do not produce a swelling that can be felt and are almost always detected at pathological examination for cancer suspected for other reasons – such as innocent fibrosis or cysts. Rarely, minimal cancers of this kind may become chalky (*calcified*) and may be detected by high-grade special X-ray examination (*mammography*).

The diagnosis of breast cancer is by microscopic examination by a pathologist, of tissue from the lump. This is called a biopsy and the tissue may be obtained by cutting into the breast and removing suspect tissue under direct inspection, or by sucking out some cells through a needle. The significance and probable outcome of breast cancer depend on the stage the tumour has reached when discovered. The size of the cancer is one of the most important factors. With tumours less than 2 cm across at the time of diagnosis and treatment, 60% of women are free of recurrences five years later. If tumours are 2–5 cm across, about 45% of the women are free of recurrence at five years. But for tumours more than 5 cm across, only about 20% of women are free of recurrence. This highlights the importance of monthly self-examination (see BREAST, SELF-EXAMINATION). Several careful studies have shown that tumour size is substantially and significantly less, at the time of diagnosis in women who practice regular self-examination.

Mammography as a screening method for breast cancer has greatly improved in reliability in recent years and the dosage of radiation has been reduced so that it is not now believed to be a hazard. Experts now believe that mammography, if properly done, can reduce the mortality from breast cancer by one-third in women over 50.

The outlook in breast cancer is worsened if the cancer has spread to the lymph nodes in the armpit, and greatly worsened if there are discernible distant outgrowths of tumour (*metastases*). Delay in seeking investigation and treatment is therefore most dangerous. Several studies have shown that women who delay for more than three months after finding a lump, subsequently proved to be cancer, have a substantially lower survival rate then those who report the problem within three months. This fact should be known to all women, and used, if necessary as a basis for protest against medical delays. You must never delay on the grounds of fright or shyness.

Women not treated at all do very badly. Conventional treatment of breast cancer has, in the past, been mainly by radical mastectomy–surgical removal of all breast tissue and the connected lymph nodes together with the removal of the underlying chest muscles (*pectorals*). As a rough approximation, the five-year survival rate has been about 50% overall. For those without lymph node involvement, the rate has been about 70% and for those with lymph node cancer, about 30%.

It has to be stated, however, that breast cancer can spread

remotely even without involvement of the glands in the armpit. This and other factors led surgeons to pay less attention to radical and mutilating operations and more to the possibility of treatment by more limited surgery combined with various combinations of radiotherapy, anti-cancer chemotherapy, hormone treatment and immune system boosting. Radical surgery is now usually restricted to total removal of the breast and lymph tissues with preservation of the muscles. This gives much improved appearance and function and makes breast reconstruction easier. In recent years there has been a trend towards even less mutilating operations and it is now common to employ a simple removal of the mass (*lumpectomy*) followed by a course of radiotherapy using linear accelerators or a cobalt-60 source.

The study of the results of such methods shows that they are no worse than those of radical mastectomy and that cancerous nodes can be treated just as effectively by radiation as by operation. A great many clinical trials have been done to compare the effectiveness of various regimes of treatment for cancer that has spread beyond the breast. But the possible permutations and combinations of different methods and different groups, in terms of cancer stage, are so great that the results are difficult to interpret. Moreover, not all present methods of cancer treatment have been available long enough for the long-term outcome to be known. We do know, however, that chemotherapy substantially reduces the mortality in pre-menopausal women with cancer that has spread to the lymph nodes in the armpit. Hormonal therapy has been found most useful in cases where the cancer has spread widely. Immune system therapy is recent and promising.

Traditionally, the treatment of breast cancer has been the province of the general surgeon. This is no longer considered appropriate. Breast cancer is a speciality in its own right calling for specialized knowledge and skills. The results of treatment by such specialists are significantly better than those of most general surgeons. This fact has recently been recognized by the British government and new guidelines for the setting up of specialized cancer centres have been published.

See also BREAST LUMP, BREAST RECONSTRUCTION, BREAST REMOVAL, TAMOXIFEN.

### Breast cancer prevention

See BREAST SELF-EXAMINATION, MAMMOGRAPHY, TAMOXIFEN.

### Breast cancer screening

See BREAST SELF-EXAMINATION, MAMMOGRAPHY.

### Breast enlargement

This may occur in both sexes during the first ten days after birth, because of the passage of maternal sex hormones into the fetal blood. In girls, the breasts enlarge at puberty under the influence of the hormones. Budding starts around age ten or eleven and breast growth progresses to the age of thirteen or fourteen. Oestrogen stimulates the growth of the ducts and progesterone the gland tissue. Progesterone also stimulates congestion of the glands during the second half of each menstrual cycle and breast enlargement occurs. This settles when the next period starts. Cancer does not cause breast enlargement in the absence of other obvious signs, such as a lump.

Breast enlargement is a normal feature of pregnancy and

may be considerable. Even greater enlargement is to be expected during milk production (*lactation*) due to milk engorgement and increased blood supply. Breast enlargement occurring during pregnancy usually settles down after the baby is weaned.

There is a great range of variation in the size of the normal breast and breasts are sometimes of different sizes. Abnormal enlargement (*hypertrophy*) may affect one or both sides and often appears at puberty. This is due to an increase both in glandular tissue and fat and the weight and stretching may cause great discomfort. Teenagers are often gravely embarrassed by over-large breasts and surgical BREAST REDUCTION is sometimes performed as a medical indication. Commercial surgery is, of course, always available.

## Breastfeeding

From every point of view except that of working convenience, breastfeeding is best for both mother and baby. The chemical and dietary constitution of breast milk is attuned to the digestive capacity of the baby and the nutritional balance is exactly what is required. Maternal antibodies to many infections are also supplied so that the baby has a valuable degree of protection to cover the period before its own immune system can take over.

At the time of delivery, the levels of the hormone prolactin are at their highest and once the afterbirth (*placenta*) has gone, this hormone is free to exert its full effect on the breasts. Prolactin production by the pituitary gland is increased by handling and touching the breasts and especially by the stimulus of suckling by the baby. Milk production is fully estab-

45

lished two to five days after delivery and the breasts become enlarged and tender. About one third of the breast size is due to the presence of milk in the glands and ducts and most of the actual synthesis of the milk occurs while the baby is suckling and the prolactin levels are at their highest. So it is essentially suckling that maintains the supply of milk and this may be continued indefinitely, as in the case of 'wet nurses' in former times.

Human milk contains fat, protein (casein, lactalbumin, lactoglobulin), sugar (lactose), vitamins (C, A and D) and minerals (sodium, potassium, calcium, iron, magnesium, etc). All these constituents are also present in cows' milk, but in such differing concentrations that it is impossible, by dilution or supplementation, to turn the one into the other. This is one reason why breast milk is always to be preferred to formula milk.

The milk secreted under the influence of prolactin must move into the ducts behind the nipple before the baby can suck and squeeze it out. The movement into the ducts is called 'milk let-down' and this is under the influence of another pituitary hormone called oxytocin. This, like prolactin, is prompted by suckling and, very sensitively, by psychological factors. A nursing mother may find that she will leak milk simply as a result of hearing her baby cry.

Breastfeeding prevents ovulation in a proportion of cases, but it should not be relied upon as a contraceptive. When nursing is discontinued for a few days, the pressure of the milk closes off the small blood vessels in the gland and, since the milk is secreted from the blood, the supply soon fails. Fat cells in the breast connective tissue often increase in size and the breasts may end up larger than before the pregnancy.

Telephone advice can be obtained from the Counselling Service of the Association of Breastfeeding Mothers, 7 Maybourne Close, London SE26 6EF. Tel: 081 778 4769.

## Breast inflammation

The medical term for this is mastitis. This is commonest during the period of milk production (*lactation*) and is usually caused by infection with germs that get in through cracks or abrasions in the nipples. Mastitis is especially likely if the baby has a skin infection. It causes high fever, local redness, pain, tenderness and hardening, and, unless the infection is successfully controlled by early antibiotic treatment, an abscess may form which may have to be opened and drained surgically.

The term *chronic mastitis* is sometimes applied to a condition in which the breasts are of an irregular rubbery consistency and contain painful or tender nodules or cysts. This is not an inflammation and the condition, which is common, is not a mastitis. It is related to the balance of the hormones which control the menstrual cycle and does not normally require treatment.

## Breast leakage

This is called galactorrhoea, which means, literally, 'a flowing of milk'. The term is used to indicate an excessive flow, or spontaneous production of milk at times when lactation should not be occurring. Milk supply can be kept up almost indefinitely if the stimulus of suckling continues, but once this is removed, lactation ceases.

Galactorrhoea can occur in both women and men and even in babies. About 30% of the cells of the front half of the pituitary gland are prolactin hormone-producing cells; a tumour of these, a prolactinoma, will secrete large quantities of the hormone and promote a flow of milk from the breasts. Unexplained galactorrhoea in an adult is thus an important sign of a possibly serious condition – a pituitary gland tumour – and should never be ignored. Galactorrhoea may also occur as a side-effect of certain drugs.

Just before birth, babies are exposed to concentrations of this hormone in the maternal blood and often show some milk production – *witches milk* – for a few days after birth. This is quite normal and harmless.

## Breast lump

All breasts are naturally lumpy as they contain glandular tissue and this normal lumpiness is often more obvious just before a menstrual period. Sometimes what seems to be a new swelling is felt before a period. Such a swelling is often tender or painful but disappears after the end of menstruation. This kind of swelling is most unlikely to be serious.

The term 'breast lump' refers to an isolated, usually painless, swelling. Such a lump, which does not become more prominent before a period and which does not disappear afterwards, should always be regarded as potentially serious and should be reported without delay. Most breast lumps – about 75% – are entirely benign and are due either to BREAST INFLAMMATION, a breast cyst, or a non-malignant breast tumour. But breast cancer *is* common and if you are in any doubt you should regard this as a reason for reporting the lump, not for delaying (see BREAST CANCER).

BREAST SELF-EXAMINATION is an obvious precaution and should be done every month. Contrary to common belief, breast cancers are often entirely painless, so you will not know you have a lump unless you feel it, or leave it to a dangerously late stage. Don't, on any account, be put off by fear. If the doctor thinks the lump is suspicious, the chances are that all that will happen is that a few cells from it will be sucked out through a fine needle. This is called a needle biopsy and is nothing to worry about. The cells will quickly be examined under the microscope. What happens after that depends on the pathologist's findings. *Never* delay reporting a breast lump. You should protest strenuously if there is any medical delay after you have reported it. Quote government policy.

## Breast reconstruction

Women who have had to have a breast removed, usually because of cancer, present quite different problems from those who simply need BREAST AUGMENTATION or BREAST REDUCTION. Here, the requirement is for the more complicated process of breast reconstruction. Today, breast cancer surgery is often less extensive than it used to be, and reconstruction operations are correspondingly easier. But radical mastectomy, in which all breast tissue and often the underlying muscles too, are removed, leaves a woman sadly mutilated. The reconstitution of a symmetrical breast, in such a case, is difficult and may involve both tissue transplantation and plastic augmentation. But women who have had to have a breast removed deserve the sympathetic attention of the surgeon, and usually get it. Most women who have lost a breast are depressed and anxious and feel sexually disadvantaged. If you have had a breast removed and are distressed by the mutilation, you should certainly see whether something can be done to help.

It is undeniably harder to get a good result, and especially a good match in size and shape, when a breast and the underlying muscles have been removed.

In reconstruction operations the difficulty is always to achieve adequate symmetry. If the other breast is large, the reconstructed breast is likely to be too small and the question then arises as to whether a reduction operation, on the normal breast, is justified. This will, of course, mean more scars and you may feel that you already have enough of those. A perfect result is impossible and you should understand the limitations of breast reconstruction. If you feel you have real doubts about the project you may be best to abandon the idea.

It is usual to defer breast reconstruction until three months to a year after the breast removal operation. The longer period is advisable if you have had radiotherapy, which interferes with sound healing and increases the chances of graft rejection. Some surgeons, however, will undertake reconstruction at the time of the original mastectomy operation.

Simple mastectomy without removal of the pectoral muscles is usually adequately dealt with by a straightforward BREAST AUGMENTATION. But if you have had a radical mastectomy, both the skin and the underlying tissue bulk must be replaced. The operation will always be performed under general anaesthesia.

The commonest and safest site from which the necessary tissue can be taken is from your back. Just under the skin of your upper back, on either side, is a thick, broad muscle. So long as the incision is made in the direction in which the muscle fibres run – sloping up towards your shoulder from the midline – a fairly large elliptical piece of skin with attached underlying muscle, together with its blood supply, can safely be brought to the front. If the blood supply is preserved, the chances of a successful graft are very high. The edges of the cut muscle and skin are brought together with stitches. The donated skin allows the necessary increase in skin area for the new breast and the muscle helps to increase the bulk. It is not feasible to remove enough muscle to produce an adequately sized breast so an additional silicone implant is used to make up the deficit.

An alternative donor site is the front of the abdomen. Here, there is usually plenty of skin and underlying fat. When this site is used an implant may be unnecessary. In some cases, using this site has the added advantage that the procedure gets rid of an unwanted abdominal bulge and helps to produce a slimmer figure. The disadvantage is that there is a greater risk that the graft will fail to take. The loss of muscle from the abdominal wall can also lead later to hernia development.

The surgeon's final problem is to produce an artificial nipple. This is also difficult and, if done, is usually deferred for about three months. The areola can be simulated by a disc of skin taken from the inside of the thigh and the remaining nipple can be split to provide nipple tissue if it is large enough. Alternatively, an ear lobe, or a disc of skin taken from elsewhere, can be used. By this stage, many women feel they have had enough surgery and prefer to use an adhesive artificial nipple.

## Breast reduction

Unduly large, heavy and pendulous breasts are not simply an aesthetic problem. They can cause difficulty in running, skin rashes from constant skin to skin contact, grooving of the shoulder skin from the pressure of bra straps and even orthopaedic problems, such as arthritis in the neck vertebrae from the constant necessity to brace back the spine. But, to many women, the most serious effect is simply the embarrassment arising from the unconcealable bulk of mammary tissue.

Abnormal breast enlargement is quite common and, as it often occurs at puberty, when the teenager may be at her most socially sensitive, may be a cause of great distress. Enlargement may also occur at the time of pregnancy and at the menopause. Some women are so ashamed of the size of their breasts that they adopt a stooping, hollow-chested posture in an attempt to minimise the apparent size. For such women, the longing to have smaller breasts may become overwhelming. The surgery they seek is called breast reduction.

This is quite a major operation. A large breast has a large skin area and the nipple position will always be much lower than desirable so the nipple and areola will always have to be moved upwards. It would, of course, be possible to raise the nipple by removing skin from the upper part of the breast, but this would mean scars in the most conspicuous place. So the method adopted is to cut right round the areola so that the nipple and underlying breast tissue can be freed to be moved up to occupy a circular hole made higher up. From this hole, two incisions are made downwards and outwards and the skin between these, and a varying amount of underlying breast tissue, are then removed from the lower part and from either side of the breast. The amount of fat and breast tissue removed will vary from a few hundred grams to two or three kilos weight of tissue, depending on the size.

With the nipple in its new position, the skin edges can be brought together. Stitches are inserted around the areola, down the centre line of skin junction and around the junction of breast and chest wall.

If possible, the nipple is moved complete with its underlying milk duct and nerve connections. But if breasts are very large, the areola and nipple may have to be completely separated and replaced as a free graft. In this case, of course, all sensory nerves and ducts will be cut and there will be no sensation, nor any possibility of later breastfeeding. This type of operation produces an anchor-shaped scar but because the ring of the anchor forms the margin of the areola and the blades are situated on the underside of the breast, the only conspicuous part of the scar is the short vertical line corresponding to the shaft of the anchor. Scars fade in time and, if the surgery has been well done and the suturing neat, there should, after a few months, be little evidence of intervention.

Many variants of this type of technique have been developed, but these general principles apply to all.

### Complications

Bleeding and blood clot (*haematoma*) formation is one of the main worries. Some surgeons remove the dressings and check for haematomas a few hours after the operation. These will always be drained but may still become infected and lead to abscess formation.

The transplantation of the nipple may interfere with its blood supply. Cases have occurred in which a nipple has been lost from resulting tissue death. Skin incisions sometimes break down and, if this happens, the scarring is likely to be more obvious than if healing occurs directly. Nipple transplantation also leads to considerable or total loss of sensitivity. Don't forget, too, that, if you get pregnant, lactation will probably have to be stopped with hormone treatment.

## Breast removal

Surgical removal of the breast is called mastectomy. This is done almost exclusively for the treatment of cancer.

Radical mastectomy, now much less often done than formerly, involves the removal of all breast tissue and breast skin, the underlying pectoral muscles and the lymph nodes in the armpit. This involves a large, elliptical cut sloping diagonally down from the armpit to the lower part of the centre of the chest.

In simple mastectomy, only the breast tissue is removed. An elliptical cut around the nipple is used and it is sometimes possible to restore a reasonably realistic appearance with an implant. The general trend, today, is to an even less radical procedure called *lumpectomy* in which only the obvious mass is removed through a short radial cut. Ancillary treatment to reduce the chances of regrowth or recurrence of the cancer is essential.

## Breast self-examination

BREAST CANCER is the commonest form of cancer in women. Contrary to common belief, it is often entirely painless. There may sometimes be vague discomfort, but usually the only sign is a slowly growing lump. So unless you or someone else deliberately looks for it, the chances are that breast cancer will not be detected until a dangerously late stage. For any woman with breast cancer the outlook depends critically on how long the cancer has been present when it is discovered.

Clinical examination by a doctor, and especially the kind of X-ray screening known as MAMMOGRAPHY, are valuable. Mammography can detect small cancers less than 1 cm across. If there is a family history of breast cancer or any other indication, or if you are over 50, regular mammography combined with frequent examination give the best chance.

No doctor can be as familiar with the normal feel of your breasts as you are, and you can with very little inconvenience carry out the examination once a month. There is really no substitute for regular monthly self-examination and if you don't do it you may regret it. If you are still menstruating, you should examine your breasts every month during the week after your period. It is normal for your breasts to be lumpy during and just before the periods and it is more difficult then to know what you are feeling. If your periods have stopped, do the examination on a particular date – such as the first day of every month.

Here is a good routine: strip to the waist and stand straight in front of a large mirror with your arms hanging loose. Check that your breasts are of exactly the usual shape, size and colour. Check both nipples for any change in their position, relative to the rest of the breast and to one another and look carefully for any indrawing or any sign of dimpling. Check for bleeding from the nipples. Gently squeeze around each nipple to see whether you can express any discharge from the nipple itself. Look at the breast contours and check especially for puckering of the skin or an appearance like orange skin. Always compare the two sides. They need not be identical – indeed breasts seldom are – but any alteration in the usual difference may be important. Raise your arms equally above your head and check the lower parts of your breasts. See whether they move up equally when you raise your arms. Look especially to see whether one seems to be tethered or held down.

Now lie on your back so that the muscles under your breasts are relaxed and feel both breasts for lumps. Some women find it easier with a folded towel behind the shoulderblade on the side of the breast being examined. Use your right hand for the left breast and your left hand for the right. Feel only with the flat of your fingers. Do not pinch the breast tissue between fingers and thumb – it will always feel lumpy if you do it this way. Work around each breast systematically, checking each of the four quadrants and the tail of the breast which points up to the armpit. This is called the axillary tail and is especially important as many tumours occur here. Don't forget to feel carefully for lumps in the armpit. Throughout, you are searching for a firm, hardish swelling which may or may not move freely. But you are also looking for any change, however slight. If you have any suspicion of anything new, report it to your doctor at once. Delay may be dangerous.

## Breech birth

See CHILDBIRTH.

## Broken veins

This term is inaccurate and misleading. The medical word for the condition, however – *telangiectasia* – is likely to tell you even less. This appearance is due to localized widening of small veins near the surface of the skin. It is one of the natural features of the ageing skin and the cause is simply loss of support of the vessels from a reduction in the amount of the skin protein collagen. In most people, the amount of collagen in the skin declines progressively with age. Telangiectasia, which is made worse by alcohol excess and undue exposure to sun and cold, is of cosmetic importance only.

A condition called rosacea, a sort of BLUSHING disorder, features widespread telangiectasia. This condition, although nothing to do with infection, responds well to regular small doses of the antibiotic tetracycline. Telangiectasia can also be caused by frequent use of steroid preparations on the skin.

Some people are sufficiently distressed by telangiectasia to submit to destruction of the affected parts of the vessels by freezing (*cryotherapy*), electrolysis, laser treatment or electrocoagulation. This may leave small scars and recurrence is likely. The laser is probably the most effective method.

## Bulimia

Bulimia is an uncontrollable, compulsive eating disorder usually affecting intelligent young women and causing them to eat large quantities of food in a very short period of time. As many as 15,000 Calories may be taken in a few hours. In spite of this, those affected are seldom overweight and most of them appear normal. In many, the weight varies at an abnormal rate, fluctuating above and below the ideal. Friends and relatives often do not suspect bulimia because the *binge eating* and the behaviour that follows are usually kept secret. Binge episodes are often triggered by mental or social stress.

Women with bulimia can't help themselves and regularly eat to the point of bloating and nausea. These binges may, in mild cases, occur only once every few weeks, and, in such cases, strict dieting, in between episodes, is enough to keep the weight down. But in other cases, the cycle takes place every day or even several times a day. These unfortunate young women have to find a private place for their activities because the binges are followed by regret and a panicky concern that the result will be a gain in weight. So they deliberately cause themselves to vomit and take purgatives, to empty the bowel and undo the 'harm'. Some young women even take drugs, known as diuretics, which cause excessive output of urine and temporary loss of weight until the resulting thirst forces them to drink and replace the deficient fluid.

The physical problems with bulimia are caused by repeated vomiting and laxative and diuretic use, which may reduce the normal acidity of the blood and upset the balance of dissolved substances even to the extent of causing muscular weakness or the state of muscular spasm called tetany. There may be persistently sore throat and heartburn from the vomited acid, and the salivary glands in the cheeks may be inflamed in a manner similar to mumps. Teeth may be badly damaged, even reduced to sharp stumps, by the repeated action of stomach acid and the knuckles may be scarred from the attempts to force the fingers down the throat to induce vomiting.

On the psychological side, up to half the cases of bulimia have features in common with ANOREXIA NERVOSA. Women with anorexia, have a distorted image of their own bodies, and in spite of the evidence of the mirror, are deeply preoccupied with becoming too fat. Most cases of bulimia, however, are caused by a less serious psychological upset than anorexia, and treatment, by specialists in the disorder, is generally more successful. Bulimia is not just a matter of self-control but is a recognized medical condition for which medical help is needed.

# C

## Caesarean section

This is an operation, often performed in a hurry, to remove a baby from the UTERUS of a pregnant woman through an incision in the front wall of the abdomen. In ancient Rome, the operation was commonly performed immediately after the death of a woman near term. Numa Pompilius (762–715 BC) passed a law requiring that the fetus was to be cut out when a woman died in labour. This became the *Lex Caesarea* and it is likely that this is the origin of the term.

Today, Caesarean section is an indispensable procedure and has become very safe. It is done whenever delay in delivery threatens the life of the baby or the mother, or when normal delivery would be dangerous for the child. Common indications for performing the operation are:

- heartbeat changes in the fetus (*fetal distress*)
- an afterbirth (*placenta*) placed near the exit of the UTERUS (*placenta praevia*)
- the appearance of the umbilical cord before the baby
- a baby that is too large for the woman's pelvis (*disproportion*)
- breech presentation
- an excessively large baby caused by diabetes in the mother
- danger to the baby from blood breakdown (*haemolytic disease of the newborn*) resulting from rhesus incompatibility

- uncontrollable high blood pressure in the mother (*pre-eclampsia*)
- failure of the UTERUS to contract properly
- bleeding (*antepartum haemorrhage*)

The operation is performed under general, epidural or spinal anaesthesia. The incision is made, vertically or transversely, well below the navel, the bladder is pushed down off the uterus and a short transverse cut is made into the lower part of the uterus and carefully deepened until the internal, fluid-filled membranes begin to bulge through. These are left intact initially and the incision is enlarged sideways, usually by pulling with the fingers, until it is wide enough to allow the baby to get out. The membranes are now ruptured and the head delivered, followed by the body. The placenta soon separates and is removed. The wall of the uterus is closed with absorbable catgut or other stitches and the abdominal wound is closed in layers.

## Calcium

It is rare for a healthy person on a normal diet to become deficient in calcium. A daily intake of 0.5 g is normally adequate. It is now accepted, however, that women at risk from OSTEO-POROSIS will benefit from a daily supplement of the mineral in the form of calcium carbonate (chalk) or calcium gluconate. A dose of 1.5 g is recommended. Extra calcium is often advised during pregnancy and especially lactation.

## Cancer phobia

See PHOBIAS.

## Cancer screening

The commonest cancers in women are those of the breast, large bowel (*colon* and *rectum*), and, increasingly, lung. Some success has been achieved in the efforts to screen for breast cancer and the results have been most encouraging. In the USA a group of 20,000 women aged 40 to 64 were checked by careful examination of the breasts and by the special X-ray test, MAMMOGRAPHY. The mortality rate was reduced by 30% in comparison with an exactly equivalent group of women who were not screened. Ten years after the trial had started, there had been 97 deaths from breast cancer in the screened group and 137 deaths from the same cause in the unscreened group. About one third of the breast cancers detected by mammography were in the early stage before they had invaded other tissues.

BREAST SELF-EXAMINATION is an important form of screening and every woman should be familiar with the signs indicating the need for immediate medical attention.

Cancers of the large bowel frequently produce very slight bleeding, not sufficient to appear as visible blood in the stools, but sufficient to be detected by a sensitive test using paper impregnated with a chemical indicator. Trials, using this method have been reported in *The Lancet* and are accepted by about half of those to whom they are offered. It is not yet quite clear whether this is a worthwhile method. Individual awareness is essential. Blackening of the stool, from the iron in released haemoglobin, frank blood in the stools, changes in the bowel habit, unexplained and severe constipation – indeed, almost any unusual feature – should alert you to the possibility that something serious may be wrong.

Regrettably, screening for lung cancer has not been a great success. This is not because the methods are ineffective. Four-monthly chest X-rays and sputum tests can detect almost 90% of cases. But the class of people at greatest risk – young smokers of the lower socioeconomic groups – have been found to be unwilling to take advantage of such screening methods. The indications are that the money would be better spent in trying to promote measures to discourage smoking.

## Cervical erosion

This is an inaccurate term that describes a raw appearance of the outer part of the neck of the UTERUS (*cervix*). In fact, the appearance is caused by a perfectly normal extension of the inner lining (*endocervix*) out on to the usually smooth and lighter-coloured covering membrane. The extension of this velvety red area on to the cervix is especially common during pregnancy when the high levels of oestrogen promote growth of the lining of the canal of the cervix. Occasionally there is a slight mucus, or sometimes bloodstained, discharge.

Not many years ago, it was common to attribute all sorts of symptoms to cervical erosion and many treatments, especially cauterization, were given. Nowadays, gynaecologists know better, and so long as a CERVICAL SMEAR TEST shows no abnormality the condition is usually ignored. Occasionally it may cause vaginal discharge or bleeding after intercourse. In these cases treatment may be needed.

## Cervical smear test

A screening test used to detect early cancer of the neck of the UTERUS (*cervix*). It was developed by George Nicholas

## CERVICAL SMEAR TEST

Papanicolaou (1883–1962), an American pathologist of Greek origin, working at Cornell Medical College, New York. Cancer of the cervix is preventable if detected at the stage known as *carcinoma in situ* or *intra-epithelial neoplasia*. At this stage the cancerous changes in the cells (*neoplasia*) have begun, but the process is still confined to the lining (*epithelium*) and has not spread deeper. The test is performed on over three million women a year in Britain and, as a result, there has been a striking increase in the number found to have these early changes.

The 'Pap test', as it is called in the USA, is an example of *exfoliative cytology* – a technique in which isolated cells are examined microscopically by a skilled pathologist and suspicious changes noted. The Pap smear is simple. The skill lies in the interpretation of changes in the cells. A metal or plastic instrument (*speculum*) is gently inserted to keep the VAGINA open and a small, blunt-edged plastic or wooden spatula is used to scrape some cells gently from in and around the opening of the cervix. These are then smeared on a microscope slide, stained and examined.

The pathologist may find signs of inflammation from *Trichomonas vaginalis* (see TRICHOMONIASIS), THRUSH, HERPES and other infections. But he or she is primarily concerned with the characteristic cell changes caused by the human papillomavirus – a cavity near the nucleus, or a doubling or unusually deep staining of the nuclear (*chromosomal*) material. These changes are present in over 80% of cases showing suspicion of malignancy. The earliest stage of possible malignant change is shown by cells with abnormal, usually enlarged, nuclei. This is called *dyskaryosis*.

Cytology is very difficult and can be done successfully

only by experienced pathologists. Because of this difficulty, the failure to detect abnormality (false negative rate), in the very earliest stage, is admitted to be 10–15%. But cytology can detect nearly all cases of established carcinoma *in situ*. These facts emphasize the importance of repeated testing, especially if you have already had an abnormal smear result. In some centres, checks have shown, unfortunately, that only about 60% of women with abnormal smears attend for follow-up.

Ideally, three-yearly screening should be carried out on all sexually active women over 35, women who have been pregnant three or more times and women who present for contraceptive advice. Women with abnormal smears are treated by cervical freezing, high-frequency cautery (*electrodiathermy*) or laser evaporation. One treatment gives a cure rate of 95%. See also CERVIX MICROSCOPIC EXAMINATION.

## Cervicitis

This is inflammation of the neck of the UTERUS (*cervix*). Most cases of cervicitis are caused by sexually transmitted organisms, especially:

- *Chlamydia trachomatis*, which causes *non-specific urethritis*
- the gonococcus, which causes gonorrhoea
- *Herpes simplex* virus, type II, which causes venereal herpes

Often, the condition causes no symptoms, but there may be a vaginal discharge and, if infection has spread more widely, sometimes pain on intercourse. The organisms concerned often also cause urinary symptoms, such as frequency and a burning pain on urination.

The condition responds well to antibiotics, but sexual partners should also be checked and treated. It is best to avoid unprotected sexual intercourse until treatment is complete.

## Cervix microscopic examination

See COLPOSCOPY.

## Childbirth

This is the process by which the baby is expelled from the UTERUS by contractions of its muscular walls. These contractions squeeze the baby downwards and pull on the cervix causing progressive opening (*dilatation*) of the neck and outlet of the uterus. Labour is divided into three stages.

### First stage of labour

This stage lasts from the start of regular pains (*contractions*) until the cervix is fully opened (*dilated*). To begin with, the contractions are minor and occur at irregular intervals, but they gradually increase in strength and frequency until they are intense and occurring every two or three minutes. The pain experienced is due to the contraction of the walls of the uterus. The first stage may last from less than an hour to more than twelve hours, depending on various factors such as the effectiveness of the contractions, the size and position of the baby, and whether the mother has had a baby before. A fully dilated cervix is about 9–10 cm wide.

Sometimes, disproportion between the baby's head and the pelvic opening prevents progress in labour and the cervix remains only partially dilated. In such cases a CAESAREAN SECTION may be necessary.

**Second stage of labour**

The second stage is the stage of actual birth and lasts from the time of full dilatation of the cervix to the completion of the delivery of the baby. Again, the times are variable and the second stage may take only a few minutes or several hours. Under proper supervision a long second stage is uncommon. The upper part of the VAGINA stretches easily but the mouth of the vagina is less easily distended and may tear as the baby's head stretches it. A tear into the anus or urine tube (*urethra*) must be avoided and often a deliberate enlargement of the outlet of the birth canal is made, by cutting with scissors, under local anaesthesia. This is called an episiotomy and it is done when there are strong indications that tearing of the tissues in an undesirable direction is likely. Such a tear can have unpleasant long-term consequences. Episiotomy is also done to make delivery easier and may be necessary if forceps have to be used.

The descending head exerts considerable pressure on adjacent structures and this may add to the pain. Contractions of the UTERUS continue during this stage but voluntary pushing by the mother is important in assisting progress.

**Third stage**

The third stage is the period from the delivery of the baby to the delivery of the after-birth (*placenta* and *membranes*). This stage is often assisted by painkillers to assist separation of the placenta and usually lasts for about five minutes. Sometimes the placenta is delivered immediately after the baby. If drugs are not used the third stage may last for 15 to 30 minutes. Sometimes there is further delay and occasionally the placenta is retained and has to be pushed out by squeezing the

UTERUS through the lax abdominal wall or even removed by putting a hand into the uterus (manual removal). Pulling on the umbilical cord before it has separated is dangerous and can invert the uterus. When the placenta is delivered, any episiotomy incision is repaired by careful stitching and the mother is checked for *postpartum* bleeding. Severe haemorrhage at this stage is a surgical emergency calling for urgent treatment.

As soon as the baby is born it is tilted head-down so that any liquid in the nose or mouth may drain out. If necessary, the passages are cleared by mouth suction through a fine, soft plastic tube. The umbilical cord is clamped, tied with thin cord or nipped with plastic cord clamps, and cut. Antibiotic eye drops are given to prevent infection and the vital signs are checked – breathing, pulse, skin colour, muscle tone and reflexes. These points are used to determine the *Apgar score* – an assessment of the baby's overall condition.

### Umbilical cord

This is the irregular, varicose-looking supply pipe which, during intrauterine life, connects the fetus to the placenta. It is 40–60 cm long, and usually arises from the centre of the placenta. It is covered with a membrane continuous with the membrane covering the placenta. The umbilical cord consists of a jelly-like substance in which are embedded two arteries and a vein. Sometimes, there is only one artery and this may be associated with an abnormality of the kidneys.

During labour, the umbilical cord may push out alongside the baby's head and may be compressed. This is an emergency, calling for an immediate Caesarean section. Sometimes the cord is found wrapped tightly around the baby's neck. After the baby is born the cord is tied off and cut about 2.5 cm from the abdomen. The stump falls off within a week or two, leaving a scar, which is known as the navel or umbilicus.

### Epidural anaesthesia

This form of anaesthesia is popular for childbirth. Although highly effective in the relief of pain, it has no effect on the contractions of the uterus or on the ability of the baby to breathe. Epidural anaesthesia is safer than general anaesthesia, especially if this has to be given urgently to an unprepared patient who may have eaten recently and who will be liable to vomit. Vomiting is a potentially dangerous complication during full general anaesthesia. In the hands of an skilled anaesthetist, epidural anaesthesia is also safer than a spinal anaesthetic in which the anaesthetic drug is injected into the cerebrospinal fluid that bathes the spinal cord.

The spinal cord is surrounded by a tough membrane called the dura mater. Outside the dura lies the epidural space between the dura and the bony canal of the spine. It is into this space that an anaesthetic drug is injected to produce epidural anaesthesia. The needle is passed into the space between two of the spinal bones in the small of the back (*lumbar vertebrae*) and a fine plastic tube is then passed though the needle so that its end lies in the epidural space. Anaesthetic can then be injected from time to time as needed.

The main snag about epidural anaesthesia is that it is difficult and requires the services of an experienced and skilled anaesthetist. It is valuable for long-term anaesthesia but reduces the amount of voluntary assistance the mother can give. Forceps have to be used more often than in deliveries without anaesthetic.

**Placental problems**

Sometimes the placenta develops in the lower part of the uterus and extends to cover the outlet so that the baby cannot be delivered normally. This is called *placenta praevia*. Any attempt at delivery would lead to dangerous bleeding and risk to the baby. Fortunately, the condition can be detected early by ultrasound and a CAESAREAN SECTION operation arranged.

During labour, or even before it, the normally placed placenta can begin to separate from the wall of the uterus. This deprives the fetus of nutrition, and delivery may become urgently necessary. Placental separation causes pain and vaginal bleeding.

**Breech delivery**

Bottom-first birth is called breech delivery. Breech presentation occurs, usually by chance, in about 3% of labours. In most cases the baby's legs are fully bent at the hips and straight at the knees so that they lie along the body. Sometimes the knees are bent so that the buttocks and feet appear together. Occasionally a leg presents.

Breech delivery is a little more dangerous for the baby than the normal top-of-the-head-first (*vertex*) delivery, and the mortality is between 2–5% in uncomplicated cases. In premature babies, the mortality, with breech delivery, is higher. The main risk is of physical damage to the baby's brain from difficult manipulation and of brain damage from lack of oxygen caused by compression of the cord during delay in delivery.

Because of these risks, breech deliveries should always be conducted in hospital by an experienced obstetrician.

If detected at an early stage, a breech presentation may sometimes be turned to a normal presentation by careful external manipulation through the mother's abdominal wall. This is done after the 32nd or 34th week and is not always free from risk. Sometimes the procedure causes separation of the placenta from the inside wall of the uterus.

**Vacuum extraction**

This is a useful alternative to forceps delivery and is used if the second stage of labour is becoming unduly prolonged; if the baby is showing signs of distress – indicating danger; or if the mother is becoming exhausted.

Vacuum extraction is done with an instrument called a *ventouse*, or *vacuum extractor*. A silicone rubber suction cup is pressed over the central part of the baby's head. This cup is connected by tubing to a vacuum pump and the air can be partially sucked out of it so that it adheres strongly to the head. A handle is attached to the cup and by means of this a gentle pull can be given in time with each contraction. In this way the baby can be safely delivered. The cost of this procedure is an unsightly but temporary and harmless swelling, or, at the worst, a large blood clot (*cephalhaematoma*), on the top of the baby's head. The haematoma absorbs within a month. See also CAESAREAN SECTION.

**Infection of the afterbirth site**

This is called puerperal sepsis – a condition which, in the days before antibiotics, often led to the death of the new mother.

The infection occurs in the raw area on the lining of the uterus, left after separation of the afterbirth (*placenta*). In the days before the nature of bacteria and the principles of infection were understood, doctors commonly proceeded directly from the postmortem room, where they had been dissecting women who had died of sepsis, to the labour ward. Hand-washing was considered neither necessary nor courteous. The women themselves were well aware of the dangers of the labour wards and would beg to be allowed to have their babies at home or elsewhere.

In 1861 Ignaz Semmelweiss of Vienna published *The Cause, Concept, and Prophylaxis of Puerperal Fever* in which he explained the carnage with perfect accuracy. The medical profession brushed his evidence aside, laughed him out of his mind and his appointment, and felt justified when he died insane. It was not until five years later, when Louis Pasteur actually demonstrated the existence and the infecting power of bacteria, that the profession, goaded by Joseph Lister, in Edinburgh, reluctantly agreed to start washing their hands. Almost immediately, the death rate from puerperal sepsis dropped from about 10% to less than 1%. With the appearance of the antibiotics in the 1940s and 1950s, childbed fever became a thing of the past.

### Death in childbirth

This tragedy is very uncommon nowadays but still occasionally occurs as a result of complications of pregnancy, or diseases aggravated by pregnancy. Puerperal sepsis, once the chief cause of maternal death, has yielded to an understanding of the nature of infection and the availability of antibiotics.

Nowadays, new mothers rarely die, but when they do it is from:

- uncontrollable high blood pressure and the resulting damage to the brain (*eclampsia*)
- severe loss of blood
- blood clots carried from the large leg veins blocking the arteries in the lungs (*pulmonary embolism*)
- severe bleeding from a pregnancy which has developed in the abdomen, outside the uterus (*ectopic pregnancy*)
- rare anaesthetic accidents
- worsening of heart disease, diabetes and some cancers

Good antenatal care can anticipate most of these possibilities and eliminate, or greatly reduce, the danger. In industrialized countries nowadays, less than one woman in 10,000 dies as a result of childbirth.

## Chlamydial infections

Infections with organisms of the *Chlamydial* genus, especially *Chlamydia trachomatis*, can cause widespread infection of the genital tract in women, and commonly lead to:

- inflammation of the neck of the UTERUS (CERVICITIS)
- inflammation and blockage of the fallopian tubes (*salpingitis*)
- inflammation of the glands that produce sexual lubricant mucus (*Bartholinitis*)

These infections are usually sexually transmitted. Chlamydia is now the commonest of the SEXUALLY TRANSMITTED DISEASES in

Britain and USA. Inflammatory blockage of the FALLOPIAN TUBES is a common cause of infertility.

## Chloasma

A mask-like area of brownish coloration, involving the skin around the eyes, nose, cheeks and forehead, which often affects women during pregnancy or when taking oral contraceptives. Chloasma sometimes occurs after the menopause. It tends to be worse if the skin is exposed to sunlight. The pigmentation usually fades in time.

## Chorionic villus sampling

Soon after fertilization, the early dividing embryo separates into two parts, one becoming the future individual and the other developing into the 'afterbirth' (*placenta*). The chorionic villi are the finger-like processes of the developing placenta which run into the wall of the UTERUS and link up with the mother's blood vessels. Since both placenta and developing fetus arise from the same two original cells, they have the same chromosomes and any genetic abnormality in one will be present in the other.

A small sample of chorionic villi can be sucked out with a syringe through a fine flexible tube passed through the VAGINA and the neck of the uterus (*cervix*) and guided to the site of the placenta under ultrasound scan viewing. Sometimes the sample is taken by passing a needle through the abdominal wall. Cells obtained in this way can be cultured and chromosome analysis done. The main advantage of this method over AMNIOCENTESIS is that it can be done as early as nine weeks of pregnancy – about seven to 11 weeks earlier. Should abnormalities be found, many mothers find it easier to accept termination at this early stage.

Chorionic villus sampling is not entirely risk-free. In about one case in 500 serious infection occurs, and the rate of spontaneous ABORTION is raised by the procedure, possibly to as high as 4%. This is about double the average rate. But that may be a small price to pay for the opportunity to detect conditions like Down's syndrome, cystic fibrosis, thalassaemia and many other conditions caused by chromosomal abnormalities in patients in high risk groups.

## Circumcision of women

This barbaric practice, illegal in Britain, causes pain, mutilation and distress to millions of women living in male-dominated societies throughout the world. It has a long history. Accounts appear in records dating back to before the time of Christ. It is practised in New Guinea, Australia, Malaysia, Southern Europe, South America, Western Asia and India, but Africa is the main location for this form of mutilation. Alleged motives vary and much is made of the claimed cultural and social importance of the act. But the real basis seems to be the desire to reduce a woman's interest in sex so that she will not be tempted to stray from her husband's bed.

The procedure may be limited to removal of the CLITORIS or may also involve radical removal of the labia minora and majora and a stitching together of the raw surfaces so that they heal across and make sexual intercourse impossible. This is called infibulation. It is done, usually between the ages of ten and fourteen, without anaesthetic. In African practice, the young woman is held down on her back by a young man who lies under her, and her legs are forced apart, by the ankles, by two others. The mutilation is performed, often by a woman, using a sharp knife or a piece of broken glass.

In enlightened societies, such practices are rightly regarded as criminal assault.

## Climacteric

The 'change of life'. The time in a woman's life after which normal reproduction is no longer possible. This is an exclusively female phenomenon and the male menopause is a magazine-writers' fiction. The term 'climacteric' is, however, sometimes applied to the general decline in sexual drive and interest experienced by some men at about the same time as the menopause occurs in women. See MENOPAUSE.

## Clitoris

This is the female version of the penis and, like the penis, is an erectile organ. It is the main centre of erotic sensitivity and has plenty of sensory nerves. The clitoris varies greatly in size from one woman to another. Its most sensitive part, the glans, or tip, is partly hooded by a fold of skin called the prepuce. This fold is connected to the labia minora. During vaginal intercourse, effective movements by the man cause this fold to massage the glans of the clitoris. If arousal is sufficient, this massage is likely to lead to clitoral erection and orgasm. Many women do not experience clitoral stimulation in this way and more direct stimulation may be needed. See also SEXUAL PROBLEMS.

## Coitus interruptus

See CONTRACEPTION.

## Colostrum

This is the yellowish, protein-rich, milk-like fluid secreted by the breasts for the first two or three days after the birth of a baby. Colostrum contains large fat globules and a high content of antibodies, and is especially valuable both for nutrition and for the control of infection in the newborn baby.

As the colostrum changes to normal breast milk, its colour changes to bluish-white.

## Colposcopy

The direct microscopic examination of the surface of the neck of the UTERUS (*cervix*). The microscope has a long focus so that it can be used well outside the vulva and the VAGINA is held open by a kind of spreader called a speculum. Colposcopy provides an excellent view of the structure of the surface lining and makes it possible to detect suspicious areas from which samples can be taken. It is, or should be, the routine next step after a CERVICAL SMEAR TEST (*Pap test*) has shown some abnormality. The Royal College of Obstetricians and Gynaecologists has recommended that, ideally, no patient with surface cervical cancer (*intra-epithelial neoplasia*) should be treated without prior examination by colposcopy.

In addition to accurate diagnosis, colposcopy offers, in some cases, the advantage of local treatment under direct visual control. Lasers or other instruments can be used, and, in the hands of experienced gynaecologists, can offer great advantages over former methods. See also CONE BIOPSY.

## Cone biopsy

The removal of a cone- or cylindrical-shaped segment of the

neck of the UTERUS (*cervix*) which includes not only the lining but also some of the underlying tissue. Cone biopsy is done under general anaesthesia when a cervical smear test has suggested that an abnormality is present and microscopic examination of the cervix (*colposcopy*) does not fully demonstrate the abnormal area. It is used when there is suspicion of pre-malignancy. Bleeding is fairly common at the time of operation and between the 7th and 10th days afterwards. This is sometimes severe enough to require readmission to hospital and even, occasionally, blood transfusion. The scarring that follows this procedure may, rarely, reduce fertility and may lead to later CERVICAL INCOMPETENCE.

There is a trend to replace 'cold knife' cone biopsy with a method using a stainless steel wire loop heated by an electric current to remove the whole of the affected region of the cervix. This operation, called the loop electrosurgical excision procedure, takes about five minutes and may be done under local anaesthesia.

## Consent

Medical or surgical treatment, or even physical examination, may be performed only with your consent. This should, ideally, be informed – that is, you should know exactly what the treatment or examination involves. In most cases the consent is implicit, in the sense that a person who consults a doctor will generally be deemed to be willing to accept that doctor's examination, advice and treatment. In the case of surgical treatment, however, implicit consent is not enough and the consent will always be recorded in writing, usually on a standard form designed for the purpose.

But you should never forget that you retain your civil rights in a doctor's consulting room or an operating theatre, and anything done to you against your will may be deemed an assault in law.

## Contraception

The very great majority of women of the Western World who are at risk of unwanted pregnancy use some form of contraception. Many of these women – about one third in the USA – rely on male or female sterilization. Another third use oral contraceptives. After that, in declining order of use, are:

- condoms (male and female)
- spermicides
- withdrawal (*coitus interruptus*)
- the diaphragm
- the cervical cap
- periodic abstinence (calendar method)
- intrauterine contraceptive devices (IUDs)

The real effectiveness of contraceptive methods is difficult to assess because apparent failures are often due to faulty use. But some methods are less liable to incorrect use than others. Including defective use, studies of British women using various methods of contraception showed that the failure rate was highest for the calendar method and then, in order of increasing effectiveness, the ranking was spermicide alone, withdrawal, condom, diaphragm, IUD, oral contraceptives, female sterilization and male sterilization. The fail rate, per 100 woman in one year, was over 15 for the calendar method and 0.02 for male sterilization.

## CONTRACEPTION

### Calendar method

This idea is based on the optimistic belief that the length of future menstrual cycles (start of period to start of next period) can be predicted on the basis of previous cycles. Egg production (*ovulation*) occurs 14 days before the start of the next period and the egg survives for about 36 hours after release. Sperms can survive for up to four days in the woman's body, after being deposited. So, if the time of ovulation were known, the days on which sperm deposition could lead to fertilisation could be identified and avoided. Unfortunately, in practice, the time of ovulation can never be reliably known, and it may commonly occur between days 12 and 16 of a 28-day cycle. This means avoiding sexual intercourse for almost half the time between periods.

For various reasons, including irregularity of the periods and uncertainty as to how long deposited sperm remain fertile, the method commonly fails. It should not be relied on unless pregnancy is secretly wished by both parties. This method is wide open to faulty use and in some series the failure rate has been almost 50 per 100 woman in one year, or, looked at in another way, an average of a pregnancy every two years.

It is widely claimed that the method can be improved by checking the basal temperature and cervical mucus. A small rise in temperature (about 0.5°C) occurs at the time of ovulation and if a rectal thermometer capable of detecting this rise is used, and a sustained rise for three days is detected, the time of ovulation may, hopefully, be determined. Around the time of ovulation, the mucus in the neck of the UTERUS changes from a thick, viscous consistency to a thin, watery quality and this, too, can help to identify the time of ovulation. Seminal fluid can be confused with watery mucus, so intercourse in the days soon after menstruation can mislead.

A combination of checking of the dates, temperature and mucus state give the best chances, but this is a lot of trouble to take for a method which is, at best, unreliable. 'Natural family planning' is the only method of contraception approved by the Roman Catholic Church.

**Spermicides**

These are available in various forms including creams, foams, jellies, pessaries and impregnated sponges. Most of them contain the surfactant nonoxynol 9 which greatly reduces the rate of movement of sperms. Sponges can be left in place for about a day without loss of efficiency. In women who have never had a baby the sponge method is said to be as effective as the diaphragm. In women with children the first year failure rate is said to be twice as high as with the diaphragm, and is nearly 30%. These claims have, however, been disputed.

Spermicides are also useful in cutting the rates of venereal infection and are known to be active against viruses. Women who use spermicides are one third as likely to get cancer of the cervix as comparable groups who do not.

**Withdrawal (*coitus interruptus*)**

This method involves the withdrawal of the penis from the VAGINA after copulation has been in progress for some time, but before the male orgasm, with its ejaculation, occurs. Coitus interruptus is a common but unreliable method of birth control which, while certainly reducing the probability of conception, by no means eliminates it. Spermatozoa can, and do, escape into the lubricating mucus produced during coitus, and semen spilled on or around the vulva is capable of causing fertilization, by sperm migration. Couples who use the method regularly are likely to find that it lets them down.

There is another sense in which coitus interruptus is a letdown. The unrestrained orgasm and the sense of release of tension enjoyed in a context of close intimacy with the partner are major elements in the quality and naturalness of sexual intercourse. Coitus interruptus precludes this blissful state and quite rightly has been proscribed since the writer of Genesis gave us his views of the matter in the story of Onan 'who spilled his seed upon the ground.'

The unhappy consequences of coitus interruptus, whether moral, psychological or theological, have doubtless been greatly exaggerated, and there is no reason to suppose that they include the spectrum of neurotic illness formerly claimed by some psychiatrists. Even so, it is a practice not to be recommended.

### Barrier methods

Condoms, diaphragms and cervical caps have the additional advantage of protecting to some extent against SEXUALLY TRANSMITTED DISEASES. This is especially true of condoms, but, to many, these are the least acceptable of the barrier methods. Condoms prevent transmission of herpes and AIDS viruses and CHLAMYDIAL INFECTIONS.

Condoms for men are thin latex rubber sheaths intended to be rolled on to the erect penis before intercourse. Most have a terminal teat to contain the semen. Condoms, used once only, seldom fail mechanically, but can fail if used without a clear understanding of their purpose – to prevent any contact between the semen and any part of the woman. The condom must be applied well before any genital contact occurs, and, after orgasm, the sheathed penis should be withdrawn before penile shrinkage (*detumescence*) occurs. The condom should be removed and disposed of, well away from the woman's genitalia. Vaseline can damage thin rubber and should not be used as a vaginal lubricant. A spermicidal jelly, or K-Y jelly, is better.

The 'female condom' is made of the same material and is a vaginal lining, wider than the male condom and with a large ring at the outer end. It has been promoted as a means of allowing women to have more control, but does not seem to have achieved the hoped-for popularity.

The diaphragm is a shallow dome of soft rubber with a covered metal spring in the outer ring and is about 7 cm in diameter. Properly fitted and inserted, it covers the cervix, acts as a container for spermicide, bars semen from entry into the UTERUS and prevents cervical mucus from entering the vagina, thus denying the normal swim channel for sperms. Spermicidal jelly is placed in the dome and the device is inserted up to several hours before it is needed. It must remain in place for at least six hours after intercourse. If a second act of coitus is imminent within six to eight hours, additional spermicidal pessaries should be used but the diaphragm should not be disturbed.

A diaphragm must be properly selected as to size by an expert and instruction must be given in the method of insertion. It is easily removed by hooking the index finger behind the edge of the forward rim and pulling gently down and out. Between use, the diaphragm should be washed and dried, inspected against a light for pinholes and stored in the container provided.

The first year contraceptive failure rate for condoms and diaphragms is between 1–4% in women over 30, but is much higher in women under 25. The diaphragm increases the likelihood of urinary infection, probably by pressing on the bladder and obstructing outflow of urine.

Cervical caps are more comfortable and can be left in place longer than diaphragms – up to 24 hours. They stay in place by suction, come in four sizes and have to be properly fitted. They are used in conjunction with a spermicide and have a first year pregnancy rate of around 10%. They should be used only by women who have had a normal cervical smear result. All women attending for contraceptive advice should be counselled about the value of regular cervical smears and offered the test, if appropriate.

**Intrauterine devices (IUDs)**

These have been in and out of favour since first introduced many years ago, and are now banned in the USA, although still used in Britain and elsewhere. Having twice been introduced and then largely abandoned, IUDs are now, for a third time, being optimistically considered. They are certainly unsuitable for many women and should not be inserted if:

- there is any question of pregnancy
- there has not been a previous pregnancy

- there has been an ectopic pregnancy in the past
- pregnancy would bring great risk to the mother
- the woman concerned has been investigated for infertility
- there is abnormal vaginal bleeding or local infection
- the UTERUS contains fibroids
- the lifestyle involves risk of sexually transmitted disease

Fitting an intrauterine device is not entirely risk-free and has caused severe fainting with critical slowing of the heart and sometimes seizures in epileptic patients. Possible local complications include perforation of the uterus and infection. There is said to be a slight increase in subsequent infertility, due to tubal infection (*salpingitis*), but this is not positively known to be due to the IUD. There may be an increased risk of ectopic pregnancy.

Some IUDs contain copper or may release progesterone. Copper-containing devices may be left in place for three or four years and probably work by promoting a low-grade inflammation in the UTERUS which prevents implantation of the fertilized ovum. Hormone-releasing devices are replaced annually. The copper-covered T-shaped plastic device has a first year pregnancy rate of 0.5 per 100 woman years. (100 woman years means 100 women for 1 year, 50 women for 2 years, 33 women for 3 years, and so on.)

The method is said to be especially suitable for women who have already completed their families and in whom there is some objection to the use of oral contraceptives.

**Oral contraceptives**
Most of these contain various combinations of the oestrogens

ethinyloestradiol and 3-methyl ethinyloestradiol (mestranol) and one of the five progestogens norethindrone, norethindrone acetate, norethynodrel, norgestrel and laevonorgestrel. The latter two are 10 to 20 times as potent as the other progestogens. Modern oral contraceptives contain very small doses of oestrogens but are every bit as effective as the earlier high-oestrogen pills. Some oral contraceptives contain progestogen only.

Studies suggest that oral contraceptives may slightly increase the risk of cancer of the cervix but do not increase the risk of breast cancer. They do, however, protect against cancer of the uterus lining and cancer of the ovaries. Oral contraceptives do not cause permanent infertility. They do not affect the rate of spontaneous abortion or chromosomal abnormalities. They do, however, increase the tendency for the blood to clot and may promote deep vein and arterial clotting (*thrombosis*). In certain circumstances this can be dangerous. They also raise the levels of blood cholesterol. Scientific studies show that women using oral contraceptives have no significantly increased risk of coronary thrombosis or stroke. Side effects also include breast tenderness, emotional upset, fatigue, skin changes including acne, nausea and weight gain.

Oral contraceptives have certain side benefits. These include less loss of blood in menstruation and less anaemia, a lowered incidence of menstrual disorders such as irregular bleeding, a reduced incidence of non-malignant breast disorders and of cancer of the uterus lining (*endometrium*). They reduce the incidence of premenstrual tension, painful menstruation, cysts and cancers of the ovaries, and, for some reason reduce the incidence of inflammation of the FALLOPIAN TUBES (*salpingitis*). They help to reduce postmenopausal osteoporosis.

Oral contraceptives work in different ways. Oestrogens counter the secretion of the follicle stimulating hormone of the pituitary and thereby prevent ovulation. Oestrogen also prevents implantation of a fertilized ovum. Progesterone acts on the cervical mucus to maintain it in the thickened state which obstructs sperm movement.

The pill is certainly effective. Various studies have given failure rates of from 0.1 per 100 woman years (one per 1000 woman years) to one per 100 woman years. For practical purposes, these figures mean that the method is almost completely successful in preventing conception.

**Other methods**

Breastfeeding is a fairly effective contraceptive. So long as it continues and there is no menstruation, the chances of having a baby are only about one in 50. It should not, of course, be relied on as a contraceptive, because ovulation occurs before menstruation.

Long-acting hormonal contraceptives can be given by injection every eight to twelve weeks and are very effective. They may cause irregular menstrual bleeding and absence of menstruation. Contraceptive capsule implants, placed under the skin, provide effective cover for five years with a pregnancy rate of less than 1%. Again, irregular bleeding may be a problem. Fertility returns soon after the capsule is removed. A silicone rubber ring, containing progesterone and oestrogen, and placed high in the VAGINA for three weeks at a time, allows regular menstruation and affords contraceptive protection as effective as oral pills.

The current status of contraceptives that reduce male fertility is uncertain as drug manufacturers are keeping quiet, at present, about the results of their intensive research. A substance called gossypol derived from the cotton plant has undergone extensive testing, especially in China, but there are doubts about its safety. This was tried after it was noticed that many men eating food cooked in cotton-seed oil became infertile. Vasectomy is, of course, highly effective.

## Cosmetic surgery

This is a branch of plastic surgery devoted to the improvement, or alteration, of the human appearance. You will find several articles on the subject in this book. See BREAST AUGMENTATION, BREAST RECONSTRUCTION, BREAST REDUCTION, DERMABRASION, EYELID SURGERY, FACE CHEMICAL PEEL, FACE LIFT, NOSE SHAPING, SCAR REMOVAL, ABDOMEN REDUCTION and XANTHELASMA.

The most commonly performed operations are those to modify the nose and the breasts. Body contour surgery by lipectomy, and other major tissue-removing procedures, tend to have a temporary effect, as does the face lift. Face chemical peel can improve the appearance of ageing facial and other skin, but, like all surgical procedures, carries some risk.

Cosmetic surgery is often legitimately sought by people whose lives are adversely affected by a conspicuous and remediable physical blemish. For these, cosmetic surgery offers a justified expedient. It cannot, however, provide a solution to deeper emotional or psychological difficulties.

## Cramps

A cramp is a minor disorder in which a single muscle, or a group of muscles, suddenly goes into a state of powerful sustained contraction. This causes severe pain which lasts until the contraction eases off. Cramp may be caused by excess salt loss from sweating and this type can be prevented by taking extra salt.

The common night cramps, which affect most people from time to time, usually involve the calf muscles. The cause has never been satisfactorily explained, but many people find that they can be prevented by taking a small dose of quinine.

Swimmers' cramp can affect the abdominal or limb muscles and sometimes leads to a panic reaction which only makes the situation worse. The best response is to tread water gently or float on the back until the spasm has passed and then to swim slowly, avoiding strenuous movements.

## Creutzfeldt-Jakob disease

A few women have developed this disease after having chorionic gonadotrophin injections for infertility. Creutzfeldt-Jakob disease is a rapidly progressive disorder of the nervous system which affects middle-aged and elderly people causing death, usually within a year of onset. Sometimes called *subacute spongiform encephalopathy*, it is an infection with a tiny protein particle called a *prion*. This is a very slow-acting agent with an incubation period of many years. It is unusually resistant to heat and to some other methods of sterilization, but can be destroyed by steam autoclaving.

The agent is known to have been transmitted by organ transplantation, neurosurgical operating instruments, and by human pituitary growth hormone injections, as well as the gonadotrophins. It is similar to the particle which causes a serious nervous system disease (*scrapie*) in sheep and *bovine spongiform encephalopathy* in cattle ('mad cow disease'). The brains of people with Creutzfeldt-Jakob disease show the same changes as are found in affected animals. The disease affects adults and is commonest in the late fifties. It takes many years to show itself, but once started, is fatal within a matter of months.

The first signs are usually irritability, fatigue, sleep disorders and neglect of personal hygiene. It soon becomes apparent that the affected person is suffering progressive dementia. Disturbance of any of the functions of the brain then become apparent. Increasing loss of memory and of intellectual function, loss of balance, paralysis, sensory loss, speech disorder, disorientation, tremor, twitching and other signs of progressive destruction of brain function occur, and the condition ends in death after a period of from three to 12 months.

There is no effective treatment. Fortunately, the chances of acquiring this dreadful disorder are very small. It affects only about one person per million of the population per year. There has been no evidence, to date, that it can be acquired by eating infected meat.

## Cystitis

Cystitis is inflammation of the urinary bladder caused by infection. This is far commoner in women than in men mainly because of the shortness of the urine tube (*urethra*) from the bladder to the exterior. You may well be familiar with the symptoms. These are:

- unduly frequent desire to visit the toilet
- getting up at night to urinate
- frequent passage of small quantities of urine
- burning or 'scalding' pain on passing urine
- involuntary passage of a small squirt of urine on coughing or laughing (*stress incontinence*)

Sometimes you might even pass a little blood in the urine, making it look 'smoky'. Occasionally, in a severe attack, there may be fever, shivering, pain in the mid-back (*loins*) and generally feeling ill.

When urine from a person with cystitis is examined, bacteria are almost always found to be present. These are commonly *coliform* organisms of a kind that normally and harmlessly inhabit the bowel. However, cystitis may be due to other germs, including those acquired during sexual intercourse such as *Chlamydia* (see CHLAMYDIAL INFECTIONS), *Trichomonas* (see TRICHOMONIASIS) and THRUSH. If you have more than very occasional attacks of cystitis your doctor will probably arrange for you to be seen by a urological specialist to check whether there is anything else wrong with your waterworks.

Most cases of cystitis can be effectively treated with antibiotics or a mixture of a sulphonamide drug and a folic acid inhibitor (Septrin). This should be rapidly effective. If not, further investigation is called for in case the infection should be of wider extent or should be connected with some other bladder or kidney problem. In menopausal women, cystitis may respond better to oestrogens than to antibiotics. This is because after the menopause the shortage of oestrogens discourages the growth of vaginal lactobacilli. These organisms produce lactic acid and this keeps other germs away. They are thus necessary for a healthy VAGINA. When the lactobacilli are not present the vagina becomes colonized by bowel organisms, especially *E. coli*. These are the commonest cause of urinary infection.

A report in the prestigious *New England Journal of Medicine* in September 1993 showed that a simple vaginal cream containing oestrogen, applied nightly for two weeks and then twice a week for eight months virtually eliminated urinary infection. The vaginal organisms were restored to the normal lactobacilli in those who were using the cream.

Cystitis can often be avoided by a few simple measures. These are:

- taking plenty of fluids to 'flush out' the urinary system
- patient attempts to continue after urination seems complete
- urination after sexual intercourse
- avoidance of nylon underwear
- no vaginal deodorants

# D

## D and C
See DILATATION AND CURETTAGE.

## Dandruff
The common scaliness of the scalp from flakes of dead skin. These scales are most conspicuous when loosened and separated by combing or brushing the hair. Some loss of surface skin cells is normal, as these are constantly being pushed to the surface by the living cells beneath. Normal standards of hair care, with regular brushing, will dispose of these. Neglect will allow the exfoliated cells to accumulate. Dandruff represents either an accumulation from hair neglect, or an increase in the normal rate of shedding, often because the skin is mildly inflamed and itchy from various causes.

One of the commonest of these is known as *seborrhoeic dermatitis*. The cause of this condition is unknown but some dermatologists believe it may be due to a yeast fungus. It is usually worse in winter and is often so mild that little is seen except scaling. It may, however, be severe, with yellowish-red, greasy, scaly patches along the hair-line and spreading to other areas of skin such as the eyelids (*blepharitis*) or the ears.

You can usually clear dandruff quickly with a special medicated shampoo, especially one containing selenium, such as Selsun or Lenium. Seborrhoeic dermatitis responds well to corticosteroid ointments, or a preparation of lithium. In some cases anti-yeast drugs are effective.

## Deodorants

The earliest deodorants were powerful perfumes which simply masked unwanted odours. Modern attempts to solve the problem of body odour rely on substances which either remove, immobilize, or chemically change odour-producing particles or prevent their production. Body deodorants contain aluminium or zinc salts and act mainly by reducing the production of sweat secretion from the glands in the armpits and groins. This sweat is called apocrine sweat and is different from sweat produced by the rest of the skin. Apocrine sweat contains organic matter that is broken down by skin bacteria to produce unpleasant-smelling compounds. An attack on the bacteria themselves can help, but antiseptics are not now approved of. The effective germicide hexachlorophene, once widely used in deodorants, has been restricted because of the danger of nerve toxicity. Daily washing and changing of clothes, supplemented, when necessary, by an underarm roll-on deodorant, is the real answer. Ecology-minded women no longer use CFC-powered aerosol sprays.

## Depression

Depression is a mood of sustained sadness or unhappiness. Numerous studies have shown that it is twice as common in women as in men. The reason for this is unknown. There is an important difference between normal unhappiness – which we all experience at times as a reaction to misfortune or boredom – and genuine depressive illness. Clinical depression involves a degree of hopeless despondency, dejection, fear and irritability out of all proportion to any external cause. Often there is no apparent cause. Associated symptoms include:

- a general slowing down of body and mind
- slow speech
- poor concentration
- confusion
- self-reproach
- self-accusation
- loss of self-esteem
- restlessness and agitation
- insomnia, with early morning waking
- loss of interest in sex

It is essential to be aware that suicide is an ever-present risk in people who are clinically depressed. Depression is especially common in elderly people. The highest incidence of first attacks occurs between the ages of 50 and 60 in women. Depression is usually precipitated by a seriously afflicting major life event, such as a bereavement, retirement or loss of status. Postmenopausal depression is often attributed to hormonal changes but there is no positive proof of this.

The causes of depression remain speculative and there are probably many. Often it seems to be the result of a damaging tendency to view oneself as being undesirable, worthless, unwanted and unloved. A depressed person often views the world as a hostile place in which failure and punishment are to be expected and suffering and deprivation inevitable. Women may be particularly vulnerable as their sexual activity and energy decline. The loss of the ability to have children, after the menopause, may add to the sense of uselessness.

It is very important to recognize true depression in your-self or in someone you know so that urgent treatment can be given. In view of the danger and distress, and since the condition can in most cases be relieved, no time should be lost in seeking medical attention. Many depressed people who could have been restored to a normal emotional and social life have committed suicide. Effective antidepressant drugs, such as the tricyclics and the monoamine oxidase inhibitors, are available. But you should appreciate that these drugs do not show their effect until about two weeks after the treatment is started.

## Dermabrasion

The passage of the years detracts from the beauty and uniformity of young skin. Evenness of skin colouring is a feature of youth and this is gradually lost as clumps of skin pigment, sometimes quite large, appear. Smoothness of surface gives way, over the years, to the cumulative effect of pitting scars from acne, chickenpox, pimples, boils and various minor injuries. Other accumulated blemishes which further damage the appearance include widened skin pores and ugly enlarged surface blood vessels. Finally, warts, moles, cysts of various kinds, skin tags and general roughness, all add their toll, so that the youthful appearance fades further and further into the background.

So, is there anything you can do to improve the appearance of the ageing skin? One answer is sandpapering. This may sound improbable, not to say brutal, but it is, in fact, a well-established method that has been used by dermatologists and plastic surgeons for years. To make it sound more clinical, the surgeons call it dermabrasion. This method was first found useful for the treatment of the very disfiguring tattooing of skin that commonly occurs in road traffic accidents, when gravel is driven into the face, or in gunshot or fireworks injuries, when the skin may be tattooed with particles of gunpowder. The method was also tried and found effective in the treatment of facial scarring from severe adolescent acne and is now quite commonly used for this. Dermabrasion has been found useful in the management of other kinds of scarring as well as fine skin wrinkles.

Some form of anaesthesia is essential and this may take the form of local injections of anaesthetic drugs or a freezing spray. In both cases, you will probably also have some sedation, as the process, however carefully done, can hardly be described as pleasant. Sometimes dermabrasion is done under general anaesthesia. The equipment is not particularly critical and machines designed for fine woodwork, with cylindrical drums of sandpaper are quite suitable. Indeed, although manufacturers of surgical equipment sell dermabrasion instruments, some surgeons prefer to use model-makers' sanding machines as some of these are kinder to the skin than the powerful, high-speed surgical equipment. Various sizes of sandpaper cylinder are used, depending on the kind of area being treated – large drums for flat areas and small for confined spaces, such as the angle of the nose. Whatever kind of equipment is used, it must have all its exposed parts – and especially the sanding drum – completely sterilized.

Dermabrasion causes quite severe bleeding because the process removes the outer layer of the skin and exposes, and ruptures, the tiny tufts of blood vessels in the deeper layers.

During the sanding, the area being treated is constantly flooded with sterile salty water (*saline*) to wash away the blood and allow the surgeon to see exactly the level being reached. If the sanding goes too deep it will remove so much skin that regeneration is impossible and severe scarring will result. One fairly small area is done at a time and, if local anaesthetic is being used, repeated injections or freezing will be required as each new area is treated.

The principle of dermabrasion is to achieve a smooth surface by sanding down any areas which are raised, even if the skin in these areas is normal. In this way, pits and depressions become relatively less deep and obvious. This process will, of course, make the skin thinner. Because a new outer layer (*epidermis*) forms over the thinned deeper layer (*dermis*), the latter remains thin. The new epidermis grows from epidermal cells lining the hair follicles and sweat glands. These extend deeply into the skin so, even if quite a lot is sanded away, the supply of epidermal cells will remain to bud out a new outer layer for the abraded skin. But if the sanding is carried so deep that all the hair and sweat tubes are destroyed, then both you and the surgeon are in trouble.

Once sanding is complete, the now raw and bleeding areas are covered with sterile dressings, such as vaseline gauze, and protected by wool and bandages. Dressings are usually left in place for several days and it may be several weeks before your skin fully recovers. Sometimes, abraded areas remain red for a very long time – even for many months – and are especially sensitive to direct or reflected sunlight. This can cause changes in colour (*pigmentation*) which may seriously detract from the good effect of the treatment. In sunny climates, this sensitivity to sunlight can be so serious that some surgeons will do this operation only in winter.

## Diabetes in pregnancy

If you are diabetic and your blood sugar control can be kept to normal during pregnancy, you will have no trouble. Unfortunately, the constantly changing situation in pregnancy makes it very difficult to achieve good control. Insulin is important to the growth of the fetus, but your insulin, whether natural or injected, does not pass through the placenta to the baby. Your blood sugar does, however, pass through and if it is high the fetus will naturally respond by producing more insulin. As a result, it stores the excess sugar in the form of fat and protein and grows larger than normal.

Over-large babies can cause problems. The baby may get to be too big for the placenta so that it is not getting enough oxygen and nutrition. It may also get to be so big that there may be disproportion between its head and your pelvis. For these reasons it is often necessary to induce labour early or have a CAESAREAN SECTION. Early delivery is always avoided if possible for the sake of the baby's safety, and every attempt is made to allow the pregnancy to proceed until at least 38 weeks. This can only be done safely if your blood sugar control has been very good.

Unfortunately, complications of diabetes may be more likely during pregnancy and complications that have occurred previously may worsen. Blood pressure, kidney problems, and particularly eye problems may occur or get worse. Regular eye checks in a specialist ophthalmic department are needed during the pregnancy.

So it is very important that you should be looked after by a hospital or a diabetic clinic, where close checks of your blood sugar, and fine tuning of your insulin dosage, are possible. Portable insulin pumps, that automatically monitor your sugar levels and automatically inject measured doses of insulin dosage, under computer control, are available. These gadgets probably offer the best way of managing pregnancy in diabetic women. But they are inconvenient and have to be permanently connected by a catheter to one of your main veins, so you may not find the idea too attractive.

Good control of your diabetes before pregnancy is also important.

## Dilatation and curettage

This simple and commonly performed gynaecological operation is usually done under general anaesthesia. The surgeon gradually enlarges the canal of the opening into the UTERUS (*cervix*) by pushing in a succession of ever-wider smooth metal rods, called dilators, until it is wide enough to admit a long instrument with a small spoon-shaped head called a curette. With this, the inside of the uterus is gently scraped, either to remove the lining in the hope of relieving abnormal menstrual bleeding, to remove any unwanted tissue or to get a specimen (*biopsy*) for examination.

After MISCARRIAGE, dilatation and curettage is often used to get rid of 'retained products of conception' – an EMBRYO that has failed to survive but has not been spontaneously expelled. The procedure was once commonly used to cause abortion in early pregnancy, but this is now usually done by suction curettage, using a fine tube.

## Douche

Vaginal douching has long been popular, especially with women with vaginal discharge. You can use plain water from a douche bag and nozzle but you must be careful to avoid the risk of infection. If you use excessive force you can drive fluid, contaminated with vaginal organisms, into your UTERUS and along the FALLOPIAN TUBES into your peritoneal cavity. This would be a disaster that would make you very ill indeed. In douching, you should avoid antiseptics, deodorants or detergents. They are likely to do more harm than good. Some women douche routinely after sexual intercourse, but this is no good as a contraceptive.

Used in moderation, douching can be helpful. But if you overdo it you can change the normal, and essential, bacterial population of your VAGINA and get reinfected with undesirable strains that can cause trouble. (See BODY ODOUR.)

## Down's syndrome

Formerly called 'mongolism', Down's syndrome is of special concern to women who become pregnant late in their reproductive phase of life. It is a major genetic disorder caused by the presence, in the maternal ovum or the fertilizing sperm, of an extra chromosome 21. Thus the affected ovum, or sperm, as the case may be, has 24 chromosomes instead of the normal 23, and every cell in the body of an individual with Down's syndrome has 47 chromosomes instead of the normal 46. In genetic terminology, it is, for this reason, known as *trisomy 21*.

The incidence of the condition varies markedly with the age of the parents at the time of conception, especially with the age of the mother. For young women, the incidence is about one in 2000. For mothers approaching menopausal age, the incidence is about one in 40. The overall incidence is about one in 700. In about a quarter of the cases, the extra chromosome comes from the father.

People with Down's syndrome have oval, down-sloping eyelid openings and a large, protruding tongue, which does not show the normal central furrow. Around the edge of the irises of the eyes, greyish-white spots are visible soon after birth, but disappear within the first year. The head is short and wide and flattened at the back and the ears are small. The nose is short and with a depressed bridge and the lips thick and everted. The hands are broad, with a single palmar crease, and short fingers, and the skin tends to be rough and dry. The stature is low and usually the genitalia remain infantile. There is slow physical development and the muscle power is weak. There is a wide gap between the first and second toes. Other congenital disorders, such as heart and inner ear defects, are common and there is a special susceptibility to leukaemia. There is always some degree of mental defect, but this need not be severe and many people with Down's syndrome are able to engage in simple employment.

Formerly, people with Down's syndrome seldom survived childhood and many died from infections. Today, those without major heart problems usually survive, but the processes of ageing appear to be speeded up and most die in their forties or fifties.

## Drug abuse

A drug is any substance, other than a food, which affects the body in any way. Drugs include tobacco (nicotine), alcohol (ethanol) and coffee and tea (caffeine). Most people are habitual drug takers and many of them are addicted to these drugs. This is not generally regarded as 'abuse' and there are many who, likewise, do not consider the occasional use of substances like marijuana (cannabis) or cocaine as 'abuse'. In many parts of the world, drugs, such as betel nut, pan or opium are used habitually and in reasonable moderation, and people doing this would not consider themselves as 'abusing' drugs. But many people do abuse alcohol and tobacco, to the detriment of their health. And there are millions who, with or without the tacit connivance of doctors, abuse drugs such as valium or librium (*benzodiazepines*), equanil (meprobamate) and many others.

So the phrase 'drug abuse' is unclear and unsatisfactory. It really means the use of any drug which is currently disapproved of by most members of a society. In an attempt to clarify the concept of drug abuse, the class of drugs used to alter the state of the mind for recreational or pleasure purposes is often divided into 'hard drugs' and 'soft drugs'. The distinction is not entirely clear, but hard drugs are those which are liable to cause major emotional and physical dependency and thus an alteration in the social functioning of the user. This group includes heroin, morphine and similar natural or synthetic substances. The soft drug group includes tranquillizers, sedatives, cannabis, amphetamines, alcohol, hallucinogens and tobacco. Classification into 'hard' or 'soft' has nothing to do with safety. The abuse of 'soft' drugs, such as alcohol and tobacco kills many times more people than abuse of 'hard' drugs.

The lucrative market in 'recreational' drugs has prompted people without social conscience, to exploit their chemical and pharmacological expertise for illicit gain. The chemistry of many of the drugs of addiction and stimulation is well known, and it is not very difficult to modify other substances so as to produce seemingly new drugs not covered by existing prohibitive legislation. These 'designer drugs' are often modifications of respectable medical products and are produced in secret laboratories without regard to their dangers, to possible unknown toxic effects or to the possibility that they may cause sterility. They can often be produced very cheaply and can be sold on the street at lower prices than existing drugs. Their manufacturers and purveyors look for legal protection from the cynical claim that they are new.

Legislators recognize that many – especially young people – are the prey of such criminals, and require protection against them. The designer drug movement is already attracting some rigorous attention. Drugs such as the fentanyl analogues (e.g. 'China white') and the amphetamine derivatives (e.g. 'Ecstasy') have already been covered by legislation in the USA.

## Dysmenorrhoea

Painful menstruation. See PERIOD PROBLEMS.

## Dysphagia

Difficulty in swallowing. It is very common to have a feeling of a 'lump in the throat' and a sense of difficulty in swallowing. This is not real dysphagia and is fairly harmless. Dysphagia is an organic disorder and may be due to a number of causes. These include:

- actual obstruction from a foreign body in the gullet
- a tumour of the gullet
- obstruction from external pressure on the gullet
- obstruction from a mass or abnormally placed structure outside the gullet
- oesophageal or pharyngeal pouch, into which some of the food passes
- a localized muscular constriction ring in the gullet
- a neurological disorder affecting the muscular contractions that control swallowing

If you have dysphagia you need urgent investigation including a barium swallow X-ray. This may show a local narrowing, or a *filling defect*, suggesting a tumour. In nervous system disorders, such as achalasia, neither fluids nor solids can be swallowed, but in tumour, fluids will often pass freely. Never neglect suspected dysphagia.

# E

## Embryo and fetus

A human body starts with a single fertilized egg (*ovum*). All the information necessary for planning the body is contained in the genetic code on the chromosomes of that egg. Half the chromosomes came from the mother, half from the father. Soon after the egg is fertilized by the sperm, it starts to split into two cells and each of these splits into two. This process goes on repeatedly, and each time the new cells take with them a perfect copy of the genetic code.

Soon the rapidly increasing number of cells are packed together into a solid sphere. The cells of this sphere continue to divide and rearrange themselves until they form a larger hollow sphere consisting of a single layer of cells only. To begin with, any one of these cells is capable of forming any part of the body. But soon, the cells at one end form a thickened layer which develops into the embryo. The other cells are used to nourish the embryo and to form the afterbirth (*placenta*).

Before long it is possible to make out a head and a tail end and the growing cell mass forming the embryo becomes suspended within the sphere by a column of cells that develops into a stalk connecting it to the region of the placenta. This stalk becomes the umbilical cord. Blood vessels develop within this stalk to connect the circulatory system of the embryo to the placenta and thus to the circulation of the mother. By now the growing cell mass is well implanted into the lining of the mother's UTERUS. Soon the main organ systems have developed and the limbs become recognizable. After about eight weeks the embryo is so obviously human that it is called a fetus.

At that stage the fetus has all the recognizable external characteristics of a human. At 10 weeks, it measures about 2.5 cm from the crown of the head to the bottom. The face is formed but the eyelids are fused together. The brain is at a very primitive state and is incapable of any meaningful form of consciousness. By three months, the fetus is about 5 cm long (crown to rump) and by four months about 10 cm long. In the sixth month, it is up to 20 cm long and weighs up to 800 g. If it is born at this stage it is unlikely to survive. Its chances increase rapidly with increasing maturity and by the time it reaches 2,000 g it would probably be able to survive outside the uterus.

During most of the pregnancy the fetus floats in a protective fluid and is surrounded by a double membrane. The fluid – amniotic fluid – has a volume of about a litre at full term. The fetus is constantly swallowing this fluid and urinating into it. Lots of cells from its skin are also released into the amniotic fluid. The placenta, at term, is a thick, disc-shaped object about 15–20 cm in diameter. Throughout most of the pregnancy, blood from the mother runs into the placenta from the uterus side and the fetal blood is pumped by its heart along the umbilical cord to the placenta. There, the two circulations come into close contact with each other but do not actually mix. Oxygen, carbon dioxide, sugars, amino acids, fats, vitamins, minerals, and maybe a few drugs, passed freely across from the mother's blood into that of the fetus. In this way the fetus is provided with all necessary supplies for maintenance as well as for body growth, and is able to get rid of waste substances.

See also PREGNANCY, CHILDBIRTH.

## Endometriosis

The lining of the UTERUS – a highly specialized, hormone-sensitive membrane – is called the endometrium. Surprisingly, uterus lining sometimes also occurs in other places. This is always abnormal and is called endometriosis. Abnormally-sited endometrium may occur in the FALLOPIAN TUBES, on the ovaries, within the wall of the uterus itself, anywhere in the pelvis, or even further afield as in the lining of the nose and the lungs. The trouble is that, wherever it may be, endometrial tissue responds to the hormones that control the menstrual cycle. It thus goes through the same sequence of changes that affects the uterus lining. Menstrual blood from the uterus endometrium escapes through the vagina, but blood produced at these abnormal sites cannot usually escape, so there is a build-up of local pressure, and pain occurs with each menstrual period.

Endometriosis of the ovary – one of the commoner sites – can eventually cause a large cyst to develop and when this is removed it is found to be full of a dark chocolate-coloured fluid. Up to half of all infertile women have endometriosis.

As you might expect, the symptoms of endometriosis disappear during pregnancy and after the menopause. So it is easy to keep them at bay by continuously taking oral contraceptives or any other treatment that suppresses the function of the ovaries. The only complete cure, however, is to have these abnormal deposits of endometrium removed by surgery.

## Endometritis

The endometrium is the inner lining of the UTERUS. Part of it is shed during the menstrual period. Afterwards it thickens up again, becomes more glandular, and develops an increased blood supply so as to be in a suitable state for the implantation and nourishment of the fertilized ovum. Inflammation of the endometrium, as a result of infection, is called endometritis. The most severe form of this is puerperal endometritis which sometimes occurs following CHILDBIRTH. Another term for this is puerperal sepsis, and, before antibiotics were developed, this was a common cause of death after delivery.

Endometritis is uncommon except after delivery or abortion because of the protection of the vaginal acidity (see CYSTITIS) and because menstrual shedding carries away infected material. Childbirth endometritis is easily treated with antibiotics. After the menopause, the barriers to womb infection are less. Menopausal endometritis features a vaginal discharge with pus and sometimes blood. These are also the signs of UTERUS CANCER, so it is imperative that they should be reported without delay. Treatment of menopausal endometritis is highly effective and may involve oestrogen therapy, minor surgery and sometimes removal of the uterus (HYSTERECTOMY).

## Erosion

See CERVICAL EROSION.

## Exercise and fitness

Exercise is natural and normal and we neglect it at our peril. But it is a mistake to think that exercise is concerned only with the muscles. No muscle can contract without an adequate blood supply to bring it oxygen and fuel in the form of glucose. Nor can it continue to contract without a good blood supply to carry away the waste products of fuel consumption. A good blood supply requires an efficiently beating heart and a good oxygen supply requires an efficiently operating air intake system – the lungs and the muscles of respiration. These three systems – the muscles, the heart and blood vessels and the respiratory system – are so intimately inter-related that it is impossible to change one without changing the others.

Your body, as a whole, is a uniquely responsive organism and will, within the limits of your heredity, modify itself so as to deliver what you ask of it. Athletes reach their level of performance by very hard work, demanding and obtaining a response from their bodies. The top athletes are not those with the best bodies, but those with the best motivation, character, determination and resolution. Your body will also very quickly drop its capabilities to a level appropriate to low demands. After six weeks in bed, it will take you a minimum of six weeks of normal physical activity to return to your former level of fitness.

The changes which occur when you make these physical demands by exertion are not simply changes in muscle bulk and power; they are changes in the heart, in the respiratory muscles, in the blood vessels, even in the brain. They are universal and their effect is widespread. Sustained exercise improves your stamina and endurance by causing enlargement and growth of small blood vessels in your muscles – including your heart – and by increasing the size and number of the energy-producing elements in the cells. These are called mitochondria. The efficiency with which you use oxygen and glucose fuel increases, and so does the amount of work your muscles, including your heart muscle, can do.

As your fitness increases, the rate at which your heart has

to beat to maintain an adequate circulation drops and your pulse gets slower, both during exercise and rest. This is because the amount of blood pumped with each beat is greater. As a result, your heart has to do less work for the same level of efficiency. You will not achieve these benefits by taking a gentle stroll once a month. Ideally, you should exercise to the point of breathlessness for a minimum of 20 minutes, at least three times a week, and the exercises should involve as many muscles as possible.

Effective exercise enables you to perform more work without using up oxygen faster than the lungs and circulation can supply it (aerobic exercise). It increases the speed with which your body recovers from fatigue. It improves the degree of attainable tension in your muscles, the ability of your muscles to utilize the fuels glucose and fatty acids in the presence of lowered insulin level in the blood, and the ability of the liver to maintain the supply of glucose to the blood, and hence to the muscles, during strenuous exercise.

All these and other factors may be involved in the changes brought about by the radical change in the pattern of activity we call training. Fortunately, these subtleties need concern only the exercise physiologist. For most women, it is sufficient to enjoy the growing sense of physical and mental well-being and the ease with which daily physical tasks are performed.

If our food intake is in excess of our fuel requirements and our fuel usage rate is low, the excess is laid down in the fat storage depots of the body and some of it is laid down in the walls of our underused arteries. Until the menopause, you are protected by your oestrogens from the number one killer of the Western world – the disease atherosclerosis. Afterwards, this can occur very quickly. Atherosclerosis clogs or closes the arteries, reduces the blood flow, causes heart attacks, strokes and gangrene of the limbs. It interferes with the most fundamental of life processes and leads to an ever-worsening capacity for work of all kinds. Exercise throughout life is one of the most important preventives of atherosclerosis.

Exercise is not just for the young. A well-exercised 60 year old should have a physical performance of about 60% of that of a reasonably fit woman of 30. Exercise is highly beneficial at every age, without exception. Well controlled trials have shown that people in their eighties and nineties become fitter and improve their performance when they take deliberate exercise. The idea that old people are incapable of exercise is a silly cultural stereotype. Exercise has also been shown to be an excellent and highly effective treatment for depression.

Doctors now appreciate that, apart from its general benefits, exercise under medical supervision can reduce the severity of angina pectoris, leg pain on walking (*intermittent claudication*) and some forms of lung disease. If you observe the three golden rules – no smoking, no overeating, lots of exercise – you can count on a substantial improvement in your health, happiness and capacity for work.

## Exophthalmos

Bulging out of the eyeballs is known as exophthalmos. The forward movement of the eyes forces the eyelids apart and causes a staring appearance. The condition is caused by an increase in the bulk of the fat and muscles behind the eye in the bony eye socket. This occurs most commonly as a result of a THYROID GLAND DISORDER. In this case the thyroid gland is affected by an immune system defect that also results in masses of antibodies and white cells (*lymphocytes*) accumulating in the fat and muscles behind the eyes. The main effect is in the six small muscles that move each eye, and the action of these is sometimes interfered with. Thyroid exophthalmos does not necessarily occur at the same time as the active thyroid disease. Eye protrusion may occur months or years after a thyroid upset. It may, rarely, even precede it.

If you have persistent and disfiguring exophthalmos and especially if there is any question of risk to your vision from pressure on the optic nerves or exposure of the corneas, you should be under the care of an ophthalmic consultant. The question of relieving the protrusion and the pressure by removing the bony floors of the eye sockets will have to be considered. There is also the possibility of reinforcing your eyelids with mersilene mesh implants.

Although thyroid problems are by far the commonest cause of exophthalmos, even if only one eye appears to be affected, protrusion of an eyeball may be caused by the presence of other material in the orbit, such as a tumour. Eye protrusion must always be taken seriously and reported without delay.

## Eyelash disorders

If you have an eyelid injury, your lashes may grow in the wrong direction because the roots have been displaced. The same thing can result from severe lid infections like septic blepharitis or the tropical eye disease trachoma. Trachoma is a CHLAMYDIAL INFECTION and can, at least in theory, be sexually acquired. Untreated trachoma scars and distorts the lid, causing the margins to turn inwards so that the lashes rub against the corneas. This is called trichiasis, and, as well as causing severe discomfort can also lead to ulceration of the corneas. Fortunately, there are highly effective treatments for trachoma. Occasionally, lashes will grow in the wrong direction for no obvious reason.

Lashes that rub on the eye can be plucked, and this gives immediate relief. But it is a short-term solution and not the best form of treatment. A plucked lash will grow again in about six weeks. Such lashes are better destroyed by electrolysis. You may have noticed that your baby's lashes turn in. If so, don't worry. Baby's lashes are so soft and flexible that they are very unlikely to cause damage to the eyes. The condition is known as *puppy-fat entropion* and it invariably rights itself without treatment. If the baby seems distressed by it, you should get specialist advice.

## Eyelid surgery

Almost all older people have suffered loss of skin elasticity. This is particularly obvious in the skin of the eyelids, which becomes lax and baggy. Youthful skin is elastic because of healthy collagen strands. Collagen is a protein which is gradually damaged by various factors, the most important being exposure to sunlight. The eyelid skin is very thin, highly mobile, and subjected to considerable stretching throughout life, so it is perhaps not surprising that, in many, the lid skin should become loose and redundant. Excess skin, which hangs down, sometimes even over the margins of the upper lids, is called *dermochalasia*.

The worst cases of bagginess are due to an additional factor – the protrusion forward of fat which has leaked through the tissue membrane which is supposed to keep it back within the bony eye socket. Such fat protrusion under the skin is called blepharochalasia. Baggy lids also occur in thyroid underactivity (*myxoedema*) and when fluid collects in the facial tissues (*oedema*) for other reasons, including kidney inflammation (*nephritis*) and allergy.

Dermochalasia is easily treated by a simple operation called blepharoplasty. This is one of the easiest of cosmetic operations and can greatly improve appearance. The excess skin can readily be picked up in a fold until the remaining skin lies snugly on the eyeball. The surplus is then simply cut off. This leaves a bare oval area which is closed with a row of tiny hair-like stitches. The scar is in the line of a skin crease and, within a week or two, is quite invisible. The operation is popular with cosmetic surgeons as it is quick, easy and highly gratifying to the patient.

Just about the only thing that can go wrong is for the surgeon to remove too much skin so that the eyes can't close comfortably and the lid margins turn outwards. This is a serious complication and is only likely if the surgeon is careless or very inexperienced.

Blepharochalasia is a different matter altogether and is much more difficult to treat. The trouble in these cases is that the fat only comes through if the retaining membrane behind the skin has become thin and weak. Even after cutting off the protruding fat and carefully sewing up the gaps in the membrane, there is a definite tendency for this form of bagginess to recur.

## Eye protrusion

See EXOPHTHALMOS.

# F

## Face chemical peel

Wrinkles are small furrows in the skin lying between ridges caused by skin laxity. The lines of the wrinkles indicate the attachment to the deeper tissue. Wrinkles are a natural feature of the ageing skin and arise from the loss of the youthful elasticity conferred by healthy collagen – the body's structural protein. The degree of wrinkling varies considerably from one person to another and this is due at least in part to damage from ultraviolet radiation from sunlight. Wrinkling is particularly common in white-skinned people living in areas of high sun intensity such as the Middle or Far East, the south-west United States, South Africa and Northern Australia.

A facelift will tighten sagging tissue but will not do much to reduce the multitude of fine wrinkles characteristic of ageing skin. Other minor skin blemishes will also persist, in spite of the tightening of the skin, and the overall result of a straight facelift may be disappointing. There is, however, an answer to this problem and, if you are sufficiently determined to go through with the somewhat daunting process of chemical peel, you may be able to enjoy what has been called *facial rejuvenation*. Note that 'chemosurgery' must never be done at the same time as the facelift. A minimum of a month, preferably two, should be allowed, following the facelift, before the skin peel is done and if you are a person of dark or olive complexion, it probably should not be done at all. You should certainly be clearly aware of what the process involves.

# FACE CHEMICAL PEEL

Skin peel is used only on the face. It should not be used on the neck as it is apt to cause scarring. The chemical used is carbolic acid (phenol), and this is a fairly corrosive substance. Different surgeons use slightly different formulae for the mixture but almost all of them use phenol made up into a soapy mixture with other chemicals including Croton oil. After your face has been very thoroughly cleansed with detergent, this mixture is dabbed on with cotton buds or other similar applicators, care being taken to press it into all the deep crevices and wrinkles. On your upper lip, the mixture is applied right to the vermilion and a little over it, otherwise there will be an obvious line around your mouth and a very unsatisfactory appearance.

As soon as the acid touches you, you will have a strong burning sensation, but phenol is so powerful that it actually anaesthetizes the nerve ending in the skin, so the pain doesn't last long. You will, however, feel it with every application to a new area. The mixture has to be put on very evenly and smoothly; uneven application causes a blotchy result. It is, of course, imperative that, when your eyelids are being done, none of it should run into your eyes. If too much is used, some will be absorbed into your body and may cause poisoning. Several studies into the toxic effects of phenol, absorbed in this way, have been done. Kidney damage can result.

As each application is made, your skin turns white, as if frozen, and then, a few minutes later, turns a dark, purplish red from inflammation. When the whole area to be treated has been dealt with, the skin is evenly stretched and is entirely covered with strips of waterproof sticking plaster. You will then have to put up with this adhesion for as long as 48 hours, keeping your face perfectly still. You will not even be allowed to talk and will have to communicate in writing. You will also have to survive on liquid nourishment sucked through a plastic tube. The worst is yet to come.

After one or two days the sticking plaster has to be removed. This process is so unpleasant that you are unlikely to be able to tolerate the torture without the use of strong narcotics. As soon as the plaster is off, the now horrible-looking surface of your face – bloody and oozing serum – is thickly covered with a reddish-brown, mildly antiseptic powder called thymol iodide. More and more of this powder is applied to the oozing surface until a thick crust has formed and it is essential that, for a further period of from three to five days, this crust should not be disturbed. So you must keep even stiller. If you were to talk or yawn widely or try to chew, the crust might fracture and the raw area might get infected, or irregular peeling, could occur. So you will just have to lie there with the crust becoming more and more uncomfortable, and with plenty of time to speculate on the ethics of cosmetic surgery.

At the end of this period the nurses will begin to apply an ointment to the crust so as to soften it, and after several more days it will be possible to lift it off. You may be shocked, at this stage, to see how red your face is, and even more despondent to learn that the redness may last for as long as three months. During this time it is essential for you to avoid exposure to sunlight, as this can seriously damage the thin, tender skin and cause a very blotchy effect. Your face may itch intolerably during this period and your surgeon may prescribe steroid ointment to reduce the irritation and redness. Local steroids will certainly relieve the itching, but they are a mixed blessing and can be harmful.

If you are the sort of person who will never tolerate any avoidable discomfort, you would do well to stay away from chemosurgery. There is no doubt, however, that this technique can improve the appearance of the skin and give an illusion of youthfulness. The phenol destroys the outer, dead, layer of the skin (*epidermis*) and even gets rid of the upper layer of the true skin (*dermis*). These layers come off with the sticking plaster. New epidermis grows, under the thymol iodide, in about a week. This new epidermis is tighter, smoother and 'younger'. The underlying layer of dermis thickens and the new skin is firm, pink, more elastic and youthful. But when the crust is removed, there is a good deal of swelling in the skin and this conceals residual wrinkles and makes your face look younger than it will be when the swelling has settled.

Once the redness has subsided, the skin will be of a lighter colour than before, and fine wrinkles and minor, superficial blemishes of all sorts, will be reduced or eliminated. Because of the lightening effect, cosmetic surgeons are rather nervous of using the method on people with dark-coloured skin, and it is easy, with such complexions, to get an uneven effect and unnatural contrasts with the untreated area.

Chemosurgery can be used, if necessary, on one small area of the face only, but this is not a good idea unless the skin is naturally pale, otherwise the contrast may be conspicuous. If used on the forehead or the eyelids, the greatest care is necessary to avoid getting the carbolic into the eyes. This accident would not necessarily cause blindness, but the outer layer of your cornea could be temporarily destroyed and the sequel to this, when the killed cells peel off, is extremely painful. You would certainly need the skilled attention of an ophthalmic surgeon.

A last word of warning. Don't be tempted to try this method on yourself. Some people have done this and ended up permanently disfigured. Even in experienced hands, chemosurgery is not entirely risk-free. The mixture used is formulated to minimize absorption so as to avoid the toxic effects. One danger is that dilution actually increases absorption. There have been one or two deaths from phenol poisoning.

## Facelift

Facelifts are usually done under general anaesthesia, but local is possible. The skin is cut through at, or preferably just behind, the hair line, and the incision extended down in front of, and close to the ears. To conceal the upper part of the incision, some hair is shaved to accommodate it. The only part of the incision that is exposed is cleverly located so close to the ear as to be practically invisible.

Working forwards and downwards from this incision, the surgeon frees (undermines) the skin and then pulls it backwards and upwards so as to tighten it and get rid of the sag and the vertical lines. This produces an overlap of skin at the line of the cut, and the redundant skin is snipped off and discarded. The undermining of the skin has to be extensive and has to be done with great care because nerves and major blood vessels must not be injured. If the operation is to succeed, the undermining must be carried forward almost to the corner of the eye and to within an inch or so of the corner of the mouth. The surgeon must take great care not to cut the skin, but must not go too deep, as to do so would risk damage to important structures, especially to the nerve twigs that supply the muscles of expression. Injury to these nerves could cause facial paralysis (*Bell's palsy*).

When the fully undermined skin is drawn back and upwards, it overlaps the ear and the line of the original incision by half an inch to about two inches on each side. Having removed excess fat, the surgeon now tacks the drawn-up skin into place with two or three stitches, making sure that the tension is just right. Too much tension may lead to hair loss. The excess skin is then cut off. Before the stitching of the new front edge of skin to the free back edge is completed, a fine, tubular soft plastic drain may be inserted on each side. These may be connected to a small pump producing gentle suction and this may be continued for one or two days. The purpose of drains and suction is to prevent the serious complication of blood clot (*haematoma*) formation under the freed skin. Haematomas cause problems such as excessive scar formation, infection and even gangrene of the skin, and must be avoided at all costs. Some surgeons rely on pressure dressings which are kept in place for about three days.

Facelifts give an improvement for up to ten years, but, in general, the older the person, the shorter the period of 'rejuvenation'. Constant abuse of flagging collagen by sun-lamps or natural sunshine will ensure minimum advantage from the operation.

## Fainting

Fainting is a temporary loss of consciousness due to a drop in the blood pressure so that the brain is deprived of an adequate supply of fuel (glucose) and oxygen. The drop in blood pressure results either from a reduction in the rate of pumping of blood by the heart or from a general widening of the arteries of the body.

Common faints usually occur from simultaneous slowing of the heart and widening of the arteries, often after you have been standing for a long time, especially in a hot environment. Such conditions impede the return of blood to the heart by the veins. A severe fright or shock may cause sudden slowing of the heart, by way of the nerves that control the heart rate. Fainting is also more likely when the volume of your blood is reduced as occurs in fluid loss from prolonged diarrhoea or excessive sweating. Low blood pressure is normally desirable, but an abnormally low degree, as in Addison's disease or from over-enthusiastic treatment for high blood pressure, can be dangerous. Fainting on taking exercise suggests heart disease.

In a faint, the vision becomes misty, the ears ring, the skin becomes pale and the pulse slow. The resultant fall is exactly what is required to restore the flow of blood to the brain, and this can be encouraged by raising the legs. The last thing a fainting person needs is to be made to sit up. Convulsions or even brain damage can result if a fainting person is unadvisedly kept upright.

## Fallopian tubes

These remarkable organs are the open-ended tubes that conduct eggs (*ova*) from the ovaries to the UTERUS. The outer, open, end of each fallopian tube has many tiny, muscular, finger-like tentacles, poised above the ovary. The inner surface of these tentacles is lined with a membrane bearing millions of fine hairs called cilia which move, like a wind-blown field of long grass, so as to waft anything small enough into the tube. At the time the egg is released (*ovulation*), these fingers sweep over the surface of the ovary, covering about two thirds of its upper surface. There is also a suction effect tending to draw material into the tube.

The ovum has to be fertilized in the fallopian tube if the timing of the development that follows is to be correct for implantation into the lining of the uterus. So the sperms have to get into the tube either just before or during the transit of the egg.

Obstruction of the fallopian tubes from inflammation from any cause results in sterility. Partial obstruction may prevent a fertilized ovum from passing on into the UTERUS. The result may be a dangerous out-of-uterus (*ectopic*) pregnancy.

The fallopian tubes are often deliberately clamped or cut as a means of permanent contraception.

## Family planning

See CONTRACEPTION.

## Fasting

Refraining from food, or sometimes food and drink, intake. In most cases, serious fasting occurs from simple deprivation or is undertaken for religious, ascetic or ritualistic reasons or to achieve some political objective. Unfortunately, those who engage in fasting are often the least well able to sustain the reduced calorie intake, while those who never fast – much of the population of the developed countries of the world – would benefit markedly. The modest fasting of Lent, Yom Kippur or Ramadan certainly does no harm and is probably beneficial to the body.

So long as water is taken, most people can fast safely for several days, living happily on their excess fat stores. If only water and essential vitamins and minerals are taken, most people could, without too much danger, reduce their fat stores to a very low level. Once the fat stores are depleted, however, the vital necessity for a fuel supply to the brain and the heart muscle results in consumption of the voluntary muscles, which soon become severely wasted so that the body is reduced to a skeletal state of emaciation. Blood proteins, such as antibodies, and those needed to maintain the water-retaining power of the blood are also consumed. The result is susceptibility to infection and water-logging (*oedema*) of the tissues.

Many people have found moderate regular fasting, say for one day a week, a useful aid to health.

## Fatigue

Tiredness may be physical or mental. Genuine physical fatigue is due to the accumulation in the muscles of the breakdown products of fuel consumption and energy production (*metabolism*). Resting for a short period will allow time for the normal blood flow through the muscles to 'wash out' these *metabolites*. In most cases, physical fatigue has a major mental element, and in many cases purely mental fatigue masquerades as physical fatigue.

Mental fatigue has nothing to do with over-use of the mental faculties. It is the result of boredom, over-long concentration on a single task, anxiety, frustration, fear, or just general disinclination to perform a particular job of work. People lucky enough to find their intellectual work absorbing may feel tired at the end of a day, but there is no persistent fatigue and the work is anticipated with pleasure.

## Fat removal

See SUCTION LIPECTOMY.

## Fetal alcohol syndrome

Alcohol is a poison to which the growing fetus is particularly sensitive. Drinking results in raised levels of alcohol in the mother's blood and this alcohol passes through the placenta to the fetus. The fetal alcohol syndrome is the group of effects on the growing fetus caused by high levels of alcohol in the mother's blood. These effects include:

- poor bodily growth giving low birth weight and poor subsequent growth
- abnormally small head size (*microcephaly*)
- facial deformity with protruding jaws and receding upper teeth
- an increased rate of congenital heart disease
- mental retardation, often with an IQ below 80
- higher fetal death rate

The death rate in the period immediately after birth is also markedly higher than in other pregnancies.

Maternal alcohol abuse during pregnancy is now recognized as being the commonest cause of drug-induced fetal abnormality. The syndrome is likely in those who drink heavily throughout pregnancy, and the severity of the effects is roughly proportional to the amount of alcohol consumed.

There is no known lower level of safety and the best current advice is that no alcohol should be taken at any time during pregnancy.

## Fetoscopy

This is a method of direct visual examination of the fetus within the UTERUS. It is done using a fine fibreoptic viewing and illumination system that is passed through the abdominal wall and the wall of the uterus into the fluid surrounding the fetus. In addition to examining and photographing the floating fetus, the doctor can take blood samples and biopsies from the fetus. At the same time samples of uterus fluid for ALPHAFETO-PROTEIN and other estimations can be taken. Fetoscopy is not, however, used primarily to obtain amniotic fluid samples.

Fetoscopy allows the doctor to confirm or eliminate suspected physical fetal abnormalities that cannot be positively identified by ultrasound scanning. It carries a slight but significant risk of causing abortion, but in cases in which there is a high probability of inherited disease or serious physical abnormality, this risk is usually considered well worth taking.

## Fibroids

See UTERINE FIBROIDS.

## Food irradiation

If food is exposed to strong ionising radiation, such as gamma rays, any bacteria and insect pests in it will be killed, and unwanted natural changes in fruit and vegetables delayed or stopped. Irradiation does not eliminate existing toxins or viruses. If the food is tightly sealed in a container, such as a polythene bag, before it is irradiated, organisms present are destroyed and no new organisms can gain access. Food treated in this way will keep indefinitely.

Food irradiation by gamma rays does not induce radioactivity, and the effects are chemical only. The main effect is the production of highly reactive, short-lived substances called free radicals which cause cell death in living organisms. Food molecules are also affected and there may be changes in flavour and some loss of vitamins.

A committee of the World Health Organisation has expressed the view that irradiation of any food commodity, up to a dose of one million rads, would present no nutritional or bacteriological hazard to the consumer. Experts from WHO point out the benefits of irradiation – the destruction of disease germs, such as salmonella in poultry; and the prolongation of shelf-life which would increase the food supply. Food irradiation is employed in nearly 40 countries, including Britain.

## Frequency

This usually means *frequency of urination* – passing urine more often than usual. This may be due to bladder irritation from infection, to excessive fluid intake, to poorly-controlled diabetes, to pregnancy, or to the use of a drug that causes excessive urinary output (a *diuretic*). Frequency of urination is sometimes of psychological origin. See also CYSTITIS, URINARY PROBLEMS.

## Frigidity

This term, with its implication of criticism of women, has

never been accepted by women, but the idea is still widely held by many men. Although some women do experience decreased libido for various reasons, frigidity is not a medical diagnosis, but an accusation levelled at some women. It is a male-oriented pejorative, implying either that the woman is short on sexual desire or interest, or cannot be turned on sexually, or have an orgasm. Implicit in the word, of course, is an unflattering comment on the sexual abilities of the man concerned, and his use of it is a predictable response to the recognition that his charms are not working.

There has always been a need for a word for the female equivalent of impotence in the male, and the term 'frigidity' is often unthinkingly used in this sense. But lack of female sexual responsiveness is not the equivalent of impotence and is, in fact, quite a different thing. Men may be highly sexually aroused but still remain limp, or may be able to perform, mechanically, although indifferent to the partner. The truth is that men and women are so unalike, both physiologically and psychologically, that there is no exact female equivalent of this common male problem. So it would be better to drop the derogatory notion of female impotence and, instead, consider why some women do not want sex or do not like it when they get it.

Often, a failure to respond sexually is merely a reflection of the very natural disinclination for sex with a man whom the woman finds unattractive. To call this 'frigidity' is simply male machismo and chauvinism. Lack of female sexual interest is often due to lack of affection – or sometimes just the expression of it – by the partner. Some men dislike the women they copulate with – one can hardly say 'make love to' – but use them to get genital satisfaction. This is really masturbation. It is not uncommon for men to use sex solely for self-gratification. Most women, on the other hand, find sex with someone they dislike distasteful. In such a situation, a frigid reaction is appropriate. Lack of tenderness, or the expression of it, can also make a woman unresponsive.

Lack of technique is not too important if the feeling is there and, in a good relationship, unless there is pathological shyness, a couple will soon work out what they want to do. Techniques should be agreed, learned and negotiated mutually. When the relationship is good, sex difficulties can almost always be overcome, but counselling, or even sex therapy, may be necessary. Other common reasons for female disinclination include:

- fatigue
- depression
- fear of pregnancy
- mourning following an ABORTION
- psychological trauma following rape

There are many gynaecological reasons for a woman's lack of sexual interest, most of them involving pain on intercourse. This is called *dyspareunia* – a word that comes from the Greek *dyspareunos* meaning 'ill-mated'. Whether this reflects historic male attitudes, or a sophisticated perception of the nature of the relationship of the sexes, is uncertain. In fact, pain on intercourse usually involves one or more organic disorder.

Conditions causing such pain include:

- a thick, persistent hymen
- inflammation of the vulva or VAGINA from thrush

- a small abscess in one of the Bartholin lubricating glands
- inflammation of the urine tube (*urethritis*)
- inflammation of the bladder (CYSTITIS)
- a tender scar from a previous episiotomy
- scars from a vaginal hysterectomy
- undue vaginal dryness

A thick hymen needs to be cut under local anaesthesia. Cystitis can cause embarrassing stress incontinence. Vaginal dryness calls either for oestrogen replacement or artificial lubrication, or both.

In addition to the causes of pain on intercourse, some commonly prescribed drugs can affect sexual interest (*libido*), directly or indirectly. These include drugs for high blood pressure, for depression and for insomnia.

### Sexual interest and the orgasm

The role of the female orgasm has been much discussed and disputed. Many deeply loving women enjoy a satisfying sex life without ever having experienced one; and male insistence on a convulsive display of the intensity of his partner's sexual feeling may often be more a matter of self-esteem than concern for his partner's satisfactions. An intense preoccupation with the female orgasm may sell magazines but has little to do with the real values of human relationships. It is, however, worth knowing something about the orgasm.

In men, the orgasm occurs at the climax of sexual intercourse, and involves a succession of spasmodic muscle contractions which cause the ejaculation of semen followed by the pleasurable release of greatly heightened muscle tension. It is rare for men to fail to achieve an orgasm. The predominant male problem is to stop it happening. The female orgasm has no reproductive function and is much less well defined than that of the male. So far as reliable information on the matter can be obtained, about 50% of women never have one. Even so, the female orgasm has received a disproportionate amount of attention, and many women, aware that they have never had a male-type orgasm, have feelings of sexual inadequacy.

The main reason for the missing orgasm in women is a failure of sexual arousal. This is usually the man's fault, but in fairness, it must be said that many women do not have orgasms even if they are highly aroused. Some writers refer to vaginal and clitoral orgasms as if these were two different things. In fact, female orgasm is always brought about by stimulation of the clitoris, but this may be direct or indirect. Vaginal stimuli are physically less directly effective, but movement of the vagina can indirectly massage the clitoris via the hood which joins the two labia minora. At the same time, there may be important psychological and emotional demands for vaginal stimulation. To many women this seems the only right thing. Direct clitoral stimulation seems unnatural and mechanical, especially if inexpert. Others need considerable direct stimulation. Many can achieve orgasm only by masturbation or by the use of a vibrator.

Usually, the female orgasm consists of one or more relatively low peaks of sexual excitement centred in the clitoris. One peak may run into another. The male-type experience – an intense peak which precludes the desire for further stimulation – is uncommon, and men should be informed of this and should not expect or demand it.

### Sex therapy

The central idea is to impose a firm agreement to indulge in plenty of slow action but with a strong veto on penetration. Sensate focus technique just means making both partners more aware of the possibilities of bodily pleasure by plenty of graded and increasingly intimate sensual massage but with no final access. A little alcohol (by mouth) and some aqueous cream (for external use only) may help. By relieving anxiety about the risk of failure, this method is especially effective for tense women and for men worried about their potency. Prohibitions – as well as inhibitions – are usually forgotten as nature eventually has her way.

### Frottage

Although this is an exclusively male behaviour, women are usually the recipients. Frottage means rubbing the body against another person, usually a stranger, for the purposes of sexual gratification. Frottage is engaged in in densely packed crowds. Without exposing himself, the male rubs his genitals against a woman's buttock or thigh.

Some frotteurs are buttock fetishists (*pygophiliacs*) but most are just sexually inadequate people who cannot achieve a more satisfactory outlet for their desires. An obvious movement away and an unequivocally angry stare will usually discourage the frotteur.

### Frustration

This is the emotion that results from the blocking of aims. Some measure of frustration is inseparable from normal life, but, for various reasons, some people suffer a much higher level of frustration than others. Chronic frustration may occur if you try to achieve goals that are inherently beyond your ability. It may also result if you seriously try for objectives that are mutually incompatible, or are equally attractive but mutually exclusive.

Frustration is extremely common in work situations. Poor working conditions, low pay and uncongenial associates may all be sources of frustration. There may be the need to submit to disliked superiors. In this situation the conflict between the desire for money and the desire to get away from a hated work situation can be a major source of frustration.

Reactions to frustration vary widely. One of the commonest is ANGER. This can make you aggressive to others, often to people unconnected with the source of the anger. Anger directed against the source may be risky, so it is displaced and directed against a safer, even if inappropriate, target. Displaced anger is a common cause of marital discord. Another reaction is to return to the methods of childhood – to withdraw into a fantasy world in which everything is exactly as it ought to be. Some people respond to frustration by the repression mechanism – they simply dismiss from consciousness any awareness of the unpleasant facts. This response is liable to cause trouble later. Repressed problems don't go away, nor do they cease to distress. Only the effects are changed, and not always for the better.

The most mature and effective reaction to frustration is to look directly at the problem, try to analyze it, and try to decide what, even at the cost of some risk, must be done to correct or at least reduce it. Frustration in one area of life is commonly balanced by achievement in another, and many mature people have found adequate consolation in this way.

# G

## Gallstones

Under the age of 40 gallstones are three times as common in women as in men. They are especially common if you are overweight. Gallstones are hard round, oval, or faceted masses of stone-like material occurring in the gall bladder or the bile duct. Most gallstones are about the size of a pea or a marble, but may be multiple and very small, like fine gravel, or so large that a single stone completely fills the gall bladder. Gallstones do not necessarily cause trouble; about 40% of people over 60 have them, usually without any indication of the fact.

Most gallstones are composed of cholesterol, chalk (calcium carbonate), calcium bilirubinate, or a mixture of these. They are more likely to occur if the composition of the bile is abnormal, if there is blockage of bile outflow or local infection, or if there is a family history of gallstones. Their presence leads to inflammation of the gall bladder (*cholecystitis*), and may block the bile duct leading to yellowing of the skin (*obstructive jaundice*) from damming-back of the bile into the blood. The passage of a gallstone down the bile duct into the duodenum is a very painful experience, known as biliary colic.

Treatment is by removal of the gall bladder (*cholecystectomy*) – done by 'keyhole' laparoscopic surgery through very small incisions, or by gallstone *lithotripsy* in which stones are shattered by concentrated sound waves.

## Genital warts

These are essentially the same as warts anywhere else in the body and are caused by the same virus, of the papillomavirus genus of the family of papovaviruses. Genital warts are often called *condylomata acuminata*, but are just ordinary warts, all the same. They are transmitted sexually. Contact with multiple sexual partners greatly increases the chances of acquiring this unpleasant condition. Because of their location they are often more exuberant and extensive than warts elsewhere. They may spread all over the labia majora. They are usually of a cauliflower-like appearance and of a pinkish colour.

Genital warts have been of special interest because of their probable association with cancer of the cervix. Some other factor is probably also involved, however. Treatment is difficult if they are extensive, and sometimes local anti-wart applications are not sufficiently effective. Surgery under general anaesthesia may be needed.

## Goitre

Goitre simply means any enlargement of the thyroid gland, from any cause. The thyroid is situated across the front of the neck just below the Adam's apple. This gland produces hormones containing iodine, and a small quantity of this is necessary in the diet. If the iodine supply is insufficient, the gland increases its activity, producing excess of the incomplete hormone, and swells up. Iodine deficiency is almost unknown in Britain, mainly because a small quantity is artificially added to table salt. Goitre was once an epidemic condition in parts of Europe.

Goitre also occurs in the condition of Graves' disease, in which the gland is overactive and there is enlargement accompanied by excessive production of thyroid hormones. This is often associated with the staring condition of EXOPHTHALMOS. Other conditions causing goitre include:

- HASHIMOTO'S THYROIDITIS, caused by antibodies to thyroid hormone
- sub-acute thyroiditis, which is probably a virus infection
- dyshormonogenesis, a genetic enzyme deficiency which interferes with normal thyroid hormone synthesis
- tumours of the thyroid gland

See also THYROID GLAND DISORDERS.

## Grief

Grief is the pattern of associated physical and mental responses to a major loss – usually to the loss, by death or separation, of a loved person. The pattern is the same, whatever the form of the loss, and varies only with the extent of the deprivation. To some, the loss of money, status or reputation may be a cause of deeper grief than the loss of a close relative or spouse; the response simply depends on the value placed on what has been lost.

The physical elements in grief are caused by overaction of the sympathetic part the autonomic nervous system. These include:

- a rapid heart rate
- rapid breathing

- restlessness and a tendency to move about
- 'butterflies in the stomach'
- loss of appetite
- a 'lump in the throat' (*globus hystericus*)

These symptoms are similar to those experienced in conditions of fear or rage, but, in the context of loss, are interpreted differently.

The psychological elements are complex and include feelings of guilt, anger, hostility, resentment, superimposed on an overall sense of pain, anguish and unhappiness. Grief follows well-marked and usually predictable stages; and there is some comfort in the knowledge that, although the practical effects of loss may persist, the severe emotional reaction to it will not. The stages include numbness, disbelief, denial, alarm, anger, guilt, consolation, adjustment and forgetting. The process may take anything from a few months to a few years.

If you are suffering bereavement it will be greatly in your interests to contact the organization *Cruse, Bereavement Care*. You can find the address of your local branch in the phone book. Cruse offers excellent counselling, companionship and sharing of grief, often from people who have, themselves, been bereaved. Cruse counsellors are experienced in all aspects of the subject, including the effects of the loss of children.

# H

## Hair excess

Excess facial hair is common in women and generally distressing. It may, ironically, be associated with thinning and greying of the scalp hair. Unnatural hairiness, of this kind, is called *hirsutism* and, if severe, it is usually regarded as a major aesthetic blemish. There is never any real problem unless the hair is visible because of its colour. Blonde or bleached facial hair is inconspicuous and generally unobjectionable.

Hair follicles are a normal feature of all skin areas except the palms of the hands and the soles of the feet. In theory, therefore, hair can grow almost anywhere on the surface of the body. Even the external skin of the nose contains hair follicles and quite luxuriant growth of hair occasionally occurs, especially in men. Whether these follicles remain dormant or spring into productive life, depends on a number of factors. The most important of these are hormonal and it is primarily the sex hormones that determine the normal variations in hairiness between men and women.

Hirsutism in women does not, however, necessarily indicate that something has gone wrong with the sex hormones. In most cases there is no medical abnormality at all and the hairiness is either hereditary, or ethnic, or just plain bad luck. If the hirsutism is severe, however, medical investigation is certainly a good idea, because a number of important conditions can cause it. Perhaps the most significant is an excess of male sex hormone caused by hormone-secreting tumours of the ovaries or the adrenal glands. This would require urgent treatment.

Hirsutism may also be due to various genetic conditions. In rare cases, chromosomal examination shows the person concerned to be of the opposite sex to that assumed. Medical treatment can cause hirsutism, especially treatment with steroids, phenytoin (used for epilepsy or trigeminal neuralgia) and streptomycin. These last two drugs interfere with the excretion of steroids by the kidneys, so that they accumulate in the bloodstream, and this may be the way in which they promote hirsutism. Some races are ethnically predisposed to hairiness and there is a genetic condition in which hair follicles become sensitized to the low levels of male sex hormone normally present in the bloodstream of women.

If, as is often the case, these factors cannot be controlled, we are left with the problem of what to do about the unwanted hair. Hairs plucked from the follicles, whether individually or *en masse* by waxing, grow to full length again in four to six weeks and the process must be regularly repeated. Shaving is easier and less painful and is almost as effective as plucking. Contrary to widespread belief, shaving does not cause hairs to become thicker and stronger. The fallacy has arisen because of what happens to the hair of adolescent males after they start shaving. But it is not the shaving that causes the toughening of the beard – simply the hormone-induced heavier growth of hair. Of course, short-shaved hairs will always feel more bristly than long hairs, and this, too, adds to the illusion.

### Depilatories

These are preparations for removing hair. Various chemicals, such as barium sulphide or thioglycolic acid salts, can soften and dissolve hairs, so that they can be wiped off, but those that are safe do not affect the follicles, and the hair grows again. Any chemical capable of softening hair is bound to be hard on the skin, so use them with care. Avoid those that cause any obvious skin inflammation.

### Electrolysis

This is a fancy name for a very simple process which removes hair permanently, but one which requires skill – and good eyesight. The word *electrolysis* means the breaking down of water into its two component gases – oxygen and hydrogen – by the passage of an electric current. It is not, however, the electrolysis that destroys the hair follicle, but rather the burning effect of the high current density at the point of application. The method is simple. You are connected to a source of electricity at low voltage via a broad pad of saline-moistened lint on which is pressed, by means of a strap, one of the metal electrodes. The other electrode is a very fine needle and when this touches your skin and the switch is closed, the circuit is completed.

The needle is pushed carefully into the hair follicle and this is most easily done using a low-powered operating microscope. When the current is turned on, the follicle is literally fried up and turns into a small scar. The current passing is registered on a milliammeter and is checked regularly. Although you may feel a strong sensation, the instrument is incapable of providing a dangerous current. The operator can tell if the application has been effective by the appearance of a small foam of gas bubbles around the shaft of the hair and by its loosening, so that it can be lifted out without the need for any force.

As only one hair can be dealt with at a time, this is clearly a tedious, time-consuming and uncomfortable business. When the foot-switch is pressed to turn on the current, you will be keenly aware of a tiny electric shock and, of course, this will be repeated many times. The operator must try to keep the current within a reasonable range, not only to avoid discomfort, but also to avoid unnecessary scarring of the skin, and this is not always easy. Sometimes a local anaesthetic is used, but this increases the risk of scarring as you will not be aware of, or object to, excessive current.

The results depend largely on the skill of the operator in placing the needle accurately and in controlling the current. If hairs are simply plucked out after inaccurate applications, they will, of course, grow again and you will have wasted your money.

Electrolysis is not all it is cracked up to be and has been condemned by some surgeons. Many dermatologists, having considered all the available methods for the removal of unwanted hair in women, have concluded that shaving (either with a good electric shaver or one of today's sophisticated double-blade razors) is probably best.

### Skin grafting

This has a very small part to play in the management of hirsutism, which is usually too widespread to make grafting feasible. Moreover, it may be very difficult to find a donor area that is not, itself, hairy. Grafting is justified in those rare cases in which the excess hair is confined to a small, localized patch. Hairy moles can easily be removed and the skin can usually be closed directly without grafting. But if they are large, a free skin graft can be taken, perhaps from behind the ear, to cover the deficit.

The commonly affected parts in female hirsutism – the moustache and beard areas – are not at all suitable for grafting. If you were able to persuade a surgeon to do this, you would probably end up looking worse than you started. It is very difficult to match the texture and colour of facial skin with skin taken from any other part of the body, and such grafts, done to cover burned or injured areas, are apt to be rather conspicuous. You will be much better to rely on bleaching and shaving.

## Hair loss

Male-pattern baldness, which starts as a receding at the temples or a patch on the vertex and progresses until it leaves only a circle of hair at the sides and the back, hardly ever occurs in women. Male baldness is of genetic origin. Baldness in either sex may also be caused by old age, disease, burns, chemotherapy or radiation for cancer and treatment with thallium compounds, vitamin A or retinoids. In toxic alopecia, the hair loss occurs some weeks after a severe feverish illness such as scarlet fever or may occur in myxoedema, early syphilis and pregnancy. Scarring alopecia may follow burns, skin atrophy, ulceration, fungus infection (*kerion*) or skin tumours.

Any drugs designed to kill rapidly reproducing cells, such as those used to treat cancer, can cause baldness. Depending on the severity of the effect, this may be temporary or permanent. Women sometimes suffer a temporary increase in the rate of hair loss after pregnancy. The effect of anxiety is difficult to assess and it is by no means certain that increased hair loss during a period of stress or special worry is due to that. Thinning of the hair is, in itself, a potent cause of anxiety.

Alopecia areata is a localized, patchy baldness of sudden onset which may affect any part of the head or body. The area affected varies considerably in extent. The cause is unknown and the outcome uncertain. The majority of cases of such baldness clear up completely without treatment, but some persist.

Much interest has been aroused, in recent years, in the possibility of curing baldness with the artery-widening drug minoxidil. This drug was introduced as a treatment for high blood pressure, but many patients taking it became hairier than desired. So the drug was tried, as a local application, for baldness. A survey in 1985 showed that 70% of American dermatologists were making up their own minoxidil preparations. It is now retailed as a solution in alcohol and propylene glycol as preparations called Regaine and Rogaine.

Minoxidil certainly encourages a fuzzy growth in people with surviving hair follicles, but it doesn't cause new follicles to grow. The treatment is expensive and must, apparently, be continued indefinitely, for there are clear indications that the new hair falls out when the treatment is stopped. See also DANDRUFF.

## Happiness and health

It is widely held that happy people are healthier and that a positive attitude, optimism, good humour and friendliness towards one's fellow creatures promotes good health. More than 100 separate studies have established, statistically, that there really *is* a positive correlation between a satisfactory and happy state of mind and good physical health. The assumption that the state of mind causes the good health has, nevertheless, been sharply criticised. Authoritative critics insist that there is no evidence that disease is a direct reflection of the mental state of the individual. No one denies that good health promotes happiness and that bad health often damages it, but it is the claim that happiness promotes health that is in question.

Unfortunately, this is a more difficult thing to prove. Happiness is an elusive concept and many people define it in terms of physical wellbeing or general satisfaction with life. People who are able to cope well with life are both happier and healthier and are often too busy looking outwards to give much time or attention to minor ailments. Pessimism and hypochondriasis go hand in hand. Behavioural psychologists have repeatedly shown that it is possible to change *dysfunctional* behaviours and attitudes and thus to improve the state of the mental health.

None of these considerations really support the view that happiness improves health. But all of them emphasize the closeness of the relationship of mind and body and the great difficulty in separating the effects of one from those of the other.

## Hashimoto's thyroiditis

This is a swelling of the thyroid gland, a form of GOITRE, that causes an ache in the neck and sometimes difficulty in swallowing. This form of thyroid gland disorder is commonest in middle-aged women and is due to the formation of antibodies to the protein from which the hormones are synthesized. These antibodies can be found in the blood, often in large quantities, and they return to the gland and attack it as if it were foreign tissue, causing inflammation and damage.

The condition responds well to administration of thyroid hormone (*thyroxine*) and this is continued indefinitely, as the gland will eventually become underactive. Steroids may also be required.

## Heartburn

A burning or aching sensation felt behind the lower part of the breastbone when a short length of the gullet (*oesophagus*) squeezes itself (spasm) or when acid from the stomach is forced up into the gullet. Heartburn is commonest after meals, especially if you have been indulging injudiciously in fatty foods. It is also worse you are lying down and acid can more easily get into the gullet. For the same reason, heartburn is common in pregnancy. It is often associated with 'waterbrash' in which bitter-tasting stomach contents come right up into your mouth.

A common cause of heartburn is hiatus hernia in which part of the stomach pushes upwards, through the normal opening in the diaphragm, into the chest.

Heartburn can be prevented by eating more wisely, more slowly and more abstemiously. See that you get proper medical attention for duodenal (*peptic*) ulceration. There have been important recent advances in the management of these conditions.

## Hip replacement

Because the high incidence of osteoporosis in women after the menopause leads to many fractures of the neck of the thigh bone, this operation has become one of the most commonly performed on women. Tens of thousands of hip replacement operations are done every year in Britain. The operation is highly successful as both the natural socket (*acetabulum*) and the natural ball, the head of the thigh bone (*femur*), are replaced. In the operation, the joint, which has been grossly damaged by loss of its blood supply or by arthritis, is completely removed. It is replaced by a plastic socket fitted into the hollow in the pelvis, and a short, angled metal shaft, which is force down into the hollow of the thigh bone, and which has on its upper end a smooth ball to fit into the socket.

The hip replacement operation is so common that you may think of it as a routine and simple procedure. This is not so. Hip replacement is major surgery, calling for great skill and substantial surgical resources. It is expensive and time-consuming. But the results are so good that, as in the case of intra-ocular lens implants for cataract, the time, trouble and cost are irrelevant.

Complications do occur, the most important being infection and loosening of the shaft of the prosthesis in the hollow of the thigh bone. The infection rate, in spite of the most elaborate precautions, is usually at least 1%. Loosening, especially after a number of years, has been a major problem and has, so far, defied the ingenuity of technology. Special bone glues are commonly used but problems of differences of elasticity between cement and bone still have to be resolved. Re-operation may be necessary in such cases. Infection may call for surgical draining and prolonged antibiotic treatment.

## Holistic medicine

The holistic movement within medicine arose as a reaction against the way technology tends to exclude human factors and relationships. Critics rightly point out that a system which manages patients in a depersonalized way, treating them as machines to be modified by drugs, is neither optimum nor particularly effective. They suggest that the doctor's function is not simply to treat a diseased organ but also to consider the patient as a whole person in his or her cultural and environmental context, with feelings, attitudes, fears and prejudices.

This is especially important of male doctors' attitudes to female patients, for it is not always easy for male doctors to envisage the special feelings of vulnerability suffered by many women when ill. For many reasons – overwork, undue preoccupation with technology, emotional poverty, fear of improper involvement – true empathy with patients is rare. This is particularly unfortunate in an age when women, while better informed than ever before of the harm that may befall them, may, at the same time, feel inadequate to enquire into, and insist on having, all the resources of modern medicine.

One hundred years ago, when doctors had at their command only a fraction of the present resources, their concern and anxiety for their patients were much more obvious than today. As a result, the reputation of the profession stood much higher than it does now. You should not infer from this, however, that doctors care less about you than they used to.

Holistic medicine has always, throughout the ages, been practised by the best of the profession; but it is right and proper, in this mechanistic age, that we should all be reminded of what this means, and of how important it is.

## Hormone replacement therapy (HRT)

Sex hormones (synthetic oestrogens) are available to alleviate immediate menopausal symptoms such as hot flushes, depression, irritability, sweating and insomnia. Doctors are generally agreed that such treatment is useful in the short term. There is less complete agreement about the longer term use of hormone replacement therapy (HRT) to treat the OSTEOPOROSIS which is so common after the menopause, and the tendency to drying up, shrinkage and infection of the VAGINA, which sometimes affects postmenopausal women. The results of many recent studies have, however, led to a progressive swing in favour of it. Decisions on HRT are, however, for you to make, and you should be in full possession of the facts.

Osteoporosis is often a serious matter, causing severe bowing of the spine or leading to fracture of the hip bone on minor physical stress (see HIP REPLACEMENT). Some women lose bone strength rapidly and these are especially at risk of the worst effects, while others seem to lose bone mass only at about the normal rate associated with ageing in both sexes. Osteoporosis causes hip fractures in about a quarter of elderly women. Women who have an early menopause are especially at risk, and HRT can largely eliminate the additional risk women suffer after the menopause. It is established that the chances of bone fracture can be halved by long-term HRT.

You should, however, understand the risks. Oestrogens alone, increase the risk of BREAST CANCER and UTERUS CANCER. At least 10 reliable studies have shown an increased occurrence of breast cancer after five years of HRT. It is difficult to get consistent figures for the increase in the risk. Of nearly 2,000 women in Kentucky who were given oestrogens after the menopause, and followed up for an average of twelve years, 49 developed breast cancer. The expected figure, for the general population, was 39, so 10 extra cases in 2,000 were, apparently, caused by the treatment. The worst reported series found an average increase to 1.6 women for every woman not on HRT. The important thing is that almost all series show that although there is an increased incidence of breast cancer, there is a *decreased mortality from breast cancer*, with greatly increased survival, among women on HRT. This important fact has led some authorities to state that fear of breast cancer is no reason to avoid HRT.

There is another reason for increased survival in women on HRT. Until the menopause, women are much less liable to heart attacks than men. This is because female sex hormones are protective against the arterial disease atherosclerosis that causes the trouble. After the menopause, the incidence of atherosclerosis rises steeply in women. HRT allows this protective effect to continue, and this has been borne out in a number of studies.

Oestrogen alone increases the risk of cancer of the lining of the uterus (*endometrial cancer*). Before the menopause, natural oestrogens are balanced by progesterone. Studies have now clearly shown that oestrogen replacement therapy combined with progesterone reduces this risk to that of the general population. There are, however, a number of snags. You are not likely to be very keen to start menstruating again. Regular bleeding also makes it more difficult to detect early bleeding from a cancer. If there is any question of abnormal or irregular bleeding you will need a DILATATION AND CURETTAGE to be sure you are safe.

Unfortunately, also, the mood improvement enjoyed from oestrogens is countered by progesterone, which may bring on a pattern identical to that of the premenstrual syndrome. If you have had your uterus removed, there is, of course, no problem and you do not need progesterone. Indeed women who have had a HYSTERECTOMY are fortunate in being able to have all the benefits of HRT with few disadvantages.

HRT causes no increase in cancer of the cervix, ovary or vulva, and worry about an increase in other cancers is unjustified. The overall mortality from all cancers in postmenopausal women taking HRT is lower than in postmenopausal women not taking HRT. Hormone replacement therapy does not increase the risk of high blood pressure, deep vein thrombosis or blood clots travelling to the lungs (*pulmonary embolism*). It reduces the risk of heart attacks and strokes.

The effects of HRT depend to some extent on the way it is given, and HRT by mouth is not necessarily best. Everything absorbed from the intestine goes straight to the liver and oestrogens are changed in the liver into a less active form. This may be sufficient to prevent the hormone from exercising its full bone-protective function. If you take your HRT by way of the skin this does not happen, as the hormone passes directly into the general circulation. Skin patches do cause their own problems, however. They can cause skin reactions and can get detached. Direct pellet implants under the skin are more reliable. This requires a minor operation under local anaesthesia every six months or so. New synthetic drugs with oestrogen action and fewer side-effects are being developed. One of these, now available, is Livial (*tibolone*).

Most doctors, although thoroughly familiar with the distressing effects of oestrogen deprivation in women, are surprisingly uninterested in long-term HRT for postmenopausal women. Only about 9% of postmenopausal women in London receive HRT for more than three years. Even women who have had their ovaries removed before the age of 30 and who are at high risk from osteoporosis as well as increased risk of heart attacks and strokes, are not offered HRT early enough to prevent these diseases. Those who know most about the matter, however, are all strongly in favour of HRT. One respectable authority, writing in the *Journal of the Royal Society of Medicine* in 1992 stated: 'Oestrogen replacement therapy is probably the most important advance in preventive medicine in the Western world for the last half century.'

## Hymen

This is the thin, perforated membrane that stretches over the opening of the VAGINA in young women and usually tears spontaneously before puberty. Sometimes the hymen is exceptionally thick, or it may even completely close off the vaginal orifice. This rare event is called imperforate hymen and requires surgical incision to allow menstrual fluid to escape. Quite often there is some hymen left at the time of the first full act of sexual intercourse. In such a case this generally gets torn and there may be a little bleeding. The notion that all virgins bleed on 'defloration' is wrong.

## Hyperhidrosis

This is the medical term for excessive sweating due to overactivity of the sweat glands. This may occur all over the skin, or may be confined to certain areas, such as the palms of the hands, the armpits, the groins and the feet. In severe cases, areas of the skin may become soggy and softened from being constantly wet. Hyperhidrosis often causes strong BODY ODOUR, as a result of bacterial breakdown of the sweat and the surface cells of the skin. This is called bromhidrosis.

The condition is usually just a variant of the normal, but may be caused by thyroid gland overactivity, fever and, rarely, a disease of the nervous system. In some cases, local hyperhidrosis is due to stress reactions or other psychological causes. It can be treated by local applications to reduce the activity of the sweat glands, or even, in extreme cases, by the surgical removal of the most active groups of glands. Many people just naturally sweat a lot, and require more than average body bathing and clothes washing. Emotional sweating usually resolves with time.

## Hyperventilation

Very deep or rapid breathing occurs normally as a feature of violent exercise. The term is, however, more often applied to a degree of deep breathing inappropriate to the oxygen needs of the body. In such cases there is excessive and abnormal loss of carbon dioxide from the blood. The result is a reduction in blood acidity. This, in turn, affects the levels of calcium in the blood, which brings about various changes in the conductance of nerves so that certain muscle groups, such as those of the forearms and calves, may go into intense spasm causing the wrists to bend and the ankles to extend.

Hyperventilation is a common panic reaction and is associated with an alarming feeling of 'not getting enough air'. It also sometimes occurs in people who feel that they are not getting enough attention. In this, the activity is usually highly successful, but is not entirely without danger. The right response is to try to persuade the affected person to re-breathe for a few minutes into a small paper or plastic bag. If this is done, carbon dioxide is returned to the blood, the blood changes are soon reversed and the drama is over.

In very rare cases, hyperventilation can be an effect of organic disease such as brain damage from infection or injury, poisoning, fever or thyroid gland overactivity. In all of these, however, there are other obvious signs of illness.

## Hysterectomy

Hysterectomy means surgical removal of the UTERUS. This can be done through the VAGINA, or, more easily, through an incision in the front wall of the abdomen. Hysterectomy is done for a variety of reasons including:

- cancer of the UTERUS
- ENDOMETRIOSIS
- large fibroids
- severely excessive menstruation (*menorrhagia*)
- excessive menstrual pain
- occasionally for sterilization

For various reasons, hysterectomy has been a very commonly performed operation in the past, especially in the USA. An estimated half a million women have a hysterectomy every year. Not so long ago about a quarter of all American women over 50 had had the operation. In Britain, hysterectomy is performed less often.

The operation may be 'subtotal', in which the body of the uterus is removed but the neck (*cervix*) is left, or total, in which the upper part of the vagina is cut around and has to be sewn closed. The latter is now the more usual procedure. A Wertheim's hysterectomy, for cancer, involves removal of the uterus, fallopian tubes and ovaries, the upper third of the vagina and all the lymph nodes in the region.

In vaginal total hysterectomy, the cervix is grasped in toothed forceps and the uterus pulled down so that the vagina is turned partly inside out. A cut is then made around the cervix and down the front wall of the vagina. This allows the surgeon to get access to the attachments of the uterus to the side walls of the pelvis, so that these can be cut and the uterus removed. The floor of the pelvis is then strengthened by stitching muscles together and the opening in the vagina is stitched closed. This approach avoids a visible scar on the abdomen, but has the disadvantage that the vaginal scars are more extensive.

After abdominal hysterectomy the vaginal scar is confined to the upper end, which becomes a blind-ended tube. No ill effects arise as a result of the slight shortening of the vagina, as this structure is very elastic and stretches easily. Sexual intercourse is best avoided for about six weeks after a hysterectomy. Any subsequent problems with sexual intercourse are unlikely to be caused by shortening or scarring, but may arise from hormone deficiency, if the ovaries have been removed.

Many women who have had a hysterectomy feel less worthy, or in some way damaged and less attractive to their partners, and it is not uncommon for women deliberately to avoid sex. Loss of libido is, of course, commonly associated with the kind of serious illnesses that have required hysterectomy. Sexual interest will, hopefully, return with recovery. Sexual problems following hysterectomy are essentially psychological and may be difficult to overcome. Psychotherapy, and especially behaviour therapy with a definite program of deliberate sexual activity, have been found to be the most effective approach. The awareness of no longer being able to bear children can add to psychological difficulties.

# I

## Incontinence

Urinary incontinence in women is far commoner than is generally supposed. Up to half of all women have experienced it and about 7% suffer regularly from this embarrassing and distressing complaint. No one wants to talk about urinary incontinence – the involuntary and undesired passing of urine. As a result, thousands of women suffer in silence. Only a third of them receive medical care or help from the social services. Incontinence is commoner in the elderly than in the young, but many young women suffer from it. Older people are more often affected mainly because the strength of the circular muscles (*sphincters*), which keep the urine tube (*urethra*) closed until voluntarily relaxed, weaken progressively with age. In addition, older women are more likely to have suffered injury to the muscles of the floor of the pelvis in childbirth. Infection of the urinary tract, also common in the elderly, is another contributory cause. There are three main types of incontinence.

## Stress incontinence

This very common form features the escape of a small amount of urine when pressure is involuntarily applied to the bladder during coughing, sneezing, laughing, weight-bearing or strenuous activity. It especially affects women who have had babies and whose urethral sphincters have been stretched. It is also commonly caused by weakening of pelvic muscles in childbirth, urinary tract infections, bladder stones or by a downward displacement (*prolapse*) of the UTERUS or VAGINA.

### Urge incontinence

More distressing is urge incontinence, in which, at a certain level of bladder internal pressure, the strong urge to pass urine is followed by involuntary and uncontrollable bladder contraction, so that it empties completely. Urge incontinence can happen at any time and during any activity, or even at rest, and is often triggered by a sudden change of position.

### Irritable bladder

This is a condition in which, for various reasons, the bladder muscle contracts intermittently, pushing out a little urine into the beginning of the urethra. As soon as this happens, the pressure of urine at this point in the urethra, causes an intense desire to relax the sphincter and pass urine. This is another cause of urge incontinence.

### Treating incontinence

The first thing the doctors have to do is to find the cause. If there is bladder infection, this must be treated. Examination of a sample of urine is necessary and often reveals the cause. X-rays, including special methods using a dye that is rapidly excreted and shows up on the plate (*intravenous urography*) will detect obstructions, stones and structural abnormalities. Ultrasound scanning can also be used. The muscle and nerve function of the bladder can be tested by measuring the internal bladder pressure. Sometimes it is necessary to examine the inside of the bladder directly by passing a narrow viewing tube called a cystoscope along the urethra. This may reveal stones, polyps or tumours.

Weak pelvic muscles can be strengthened by pelvic floor exercises and these can help to restore sphincter function.

Occasionally, surgical tightening of the muscles may be needed. In extreme cases, an artificial sphincter, that can be controlled from the outside, can be implanted around the urethra. Rarely, the solution may be to bypass the bladder altogether.

While, obviously, treatment and cure is best, many affected women prefer to use special incontinence clothing or urine collecting devices. Self-catheterization, to keep the bladder empty by draining it through a tube, is a possibility in some cases. For irritable bladder, drugs are sometimes used to relax the bladder muscle.

### Faecal incontinence

Ironically, inability to retain faeces in the rectum is usually caused by chronic constipation. The faeces become hardened and cause irritation to the rectal lining with increased peristaltic effort. As a result, fluid and small faeces are involuntarily forced out. Proper management of the constipation – high fibre intake, suppositories of glycerol or mild laxative drugs, or softening and bulking agents – will cure this type of incontinence.

Less commonly, faecal incontinence may result from:

- organic disorder – injury to the anal canal muscles from a tear during childbirth
- neurological problems such as paraplegia or multiple sclerosis
- organic brain syndrome
- dementia

In some of these cases, faecal incontinence can be avoided by the use of regular enemas to keep the rectum empty.

## Infertility

If everything is working properly in both you and your partner and you are having sex at least twice a week, you can expect to get pregnant within a few months of starting to try for a baby. If nothing happens for a year, you will have to assume that there is some degree of infertility. About 10% of couples have this problem. Fertility is not much affected by your general health or nutrition. But if you diet too strictly your periods may stop and there will be no ovulation. Very enthusiastic athletic training may also prevent ovulation. The same goes for underactivity of the thyroid gland and badly controlled diabetes.

A review of the menstrual cycle and ovulation would be helpful at this point. Between the start of the bleeding in one cycle and the start of the next, the time, on average, is 28 days. But periods may be as short as 21 days, or, in extreme cases, as long as 60. This cycle is controlled by hormones from the pituitary gland which is an outgrowth of the brain. The follicle-stimulating hormone (FSH) from the pituitary gland acts on one of the ovaries to cause a collection of cells, containing an egg, to develop. This nest of cells is called a Graafian follicle. During the first half of the menstrual cycle the Graafian follicle produces increasing amounts of oestrogen hormone. This hormone causes thickening of the lining of the UTERUS and an increase in its blood vessels and mucus glands.

In the middle of the cycle the egg is released from the follicle in the ovary. This is called ovulation. But the follicle has not yet fully served its purpose. The cells of the empty follicle develop into a mass called the *corpus luteum*, which begins to secrete progesterone, a hormone necessary to maintain the lining of the uterus so that it is suitable to support a pregnancy. If the ovum is not fertilized, the corpus luteum degenerates and progesterone production drops off. This causes the lining of the uterus to be discarded as menstruation, about 14 days after the time of ovulation.

The vaginal blood loss that occurs when the body's level of progesterone or oestrogen hormones drops suddenly is called withdrawal bleeding. Normal menstruation is preceded by withdrawal of both oestrogen and progesterone. Similar withdrawal bleeding occurs at the end of each cycle of combined oral contraceptive pills, but is usually shorter and lighter. It is the withdrawal of progesterone that produces the blood loss.

The release of an egg from the ovary is called ovulation. A released egg is swept into the FALLOPIAN TUBE and carried along towards the uterus. While in the tube, it may be met by sperms (*spermatozoa*). If not, the egg is simply discarded during the next menstruation. If pregnancy does occur, the placenta, almost as soon as it is established, begins to secrete a hormone that keeps the corpus luteum going so that the supply of progesterone is maintained for the first three months or so. After that, the placenta takes over the oestrogen and progesterone production, so that no further ovulation or menstruation occurs during the remainder of the pregnancy.

Even if you are ovulating, this may happen infrequently enough to prevent conception by sheer accident of timing. Irregular, unpredictable and infrequent egg production will, of course, reduce the chance of the egg and sperm meeting. Various tests can be done to check whether you are ovulating. If not, you can have hormones or other drugs to stimulate ovulation, or prevent it from being inhibited. The main drugs used are anti-oestrogens such as clomiphene or TAMOXIFEN. Some of these drugs are so effective that infertile couples surprise everyone by producing twins. Another method is to give 'pulsed' doses of a hormone called gonadotrophin releasing hormone. This prompts the pituitary gland to produce the hormones that cause ovulation. Other drugs used are human menopausal gonadotrophin (HMG) and human chorionic gonadotrophin (HCG). These can cause multiple pregnancies unless the hormone levels are carefully monitored.

Tests for ovulation include the measurement of blood progesterone levels, which rise in the second half of the cycle, as well as examination of the mucus in the cervix which changes at ovulation. Sometimes the pain on ovulation ('*mittelschmerz*') is severe and positive enough to indicate what is happening. In general, regular menstruation suggests that ovulation is occurring.

Infertility is commonly caused by mechanical blockage of the fallopian tubes, so that the egg and sperms are kept apart. This is almost always the result of infection. This is commonly the result of a SEXUALLY TRANSMITTED DISEASE but may also follow the normal delivery of a baby or an abortion. Pelvic infection can also result from a burst inflamed appendix or tuberculosis. The state of your fallopian tubes can be investigated by injecting a harmless dye through the cervix. If the tubes are clear the dye will pass through the outer open ends of the tubes and can be observed through a narrow optical instrument called a laparoscope. This is passed through the abdominal wall. Laparoscopy also lets the doctor inspect your tubes for visible abnormalities and your ovaries for the presence of a Graafian follicles or a corpus luteum. Blocked tubes can sometimes be reopened, but this is difficult.

Before you are put through all this, however, your partner must have a sperm count. This is easy and quick and is always done before the female investigation. Male infertility is almost entirely a question of the sperm count and whether the sperms are normal and sufficiently active. If there are no sperms in the semen there is no possibility of fertilization. The masturbation specimen should have a volume of 2–6 ml and should contain 20,000,000 sperms per ml. More than 40% of these should be energetically motile and fewer than 30% should have an abnormal appearance. It's worth remembering that long-term alcohol excess causes a low sperm count and that this usually comes back to normal if drinking is moderated. In some cases of low sperm count, treatment with synthetic male sex hormones is effective.

**Artificial insemination**

If the problem is in the sperms or is due to impotence or other failure of normal sexual intercourse, you might want to consider artificial insemination. This is very simple and you can easily do it yourself, or get your partner to do it. A quantity of fresh seminal fluid donated by your husband (AIH), your partner (AIP) or by an anonymous donor (AID) is sucked up into a narrow syringe or pipette and injected high into the VAGINA or even into the mucus in the cervix. Impotent husbands can usually provide semen by masturbation. Of course, you have to time the procedure to coincide with the period in the menstrual cycle when ovulation is most likely. This usually occurs 14 days before the next period would have started.

So you can estimate the best time on the basis of your usual cycle. Assuming no other reasons for infertility, the success rate is as high as in couples without such specific problems.

### Sperm donation

Since the 1940s, human seminal fluid has been preserved, for indefinite periods, frozen in a glycerol cryoprotectant. Sperm is stored in phials, or plastic straws, in liquid nitrogen sperm banks. Sperm donation is used in cases of male sterility, dominant genetic disease and recessive disease where both husband and wife carry the gene. Banked semen is simply thawed, sucked up into a fine syringe and injected. Fresh semen can also be used, and this is produced, by masturbation, within a few hours of use. The insemination may be done in a doctor's surgery, in a sperm centre, or in your own home.

Unless the husband's or partner's semen is used, donors are nearly always anonymous. In Britain, many of them are medical students. Whoever is the donor, elaborate precautions are taken to ensure complete screening against AIDS and hepatitis B. The largest sperm bank is the Centre d'Etude et de Conservation du Sperm Humain (CECOS) in France. There, donors are asked to give one, two or three ejaculates a week for a month and then never again. The plastic straws in which the semen is stored each contain enough for one insemination, and a liberal supplier can fill over two hundred of these straws.

A child born from fertilization by donated sperm is deemed, by a legal presumption, to be the legitimate child of the husband. Since the procedure involves no sexual act, it is not generally considered adultery, but the Roman Catholic church has reservations.

### *In vitro* fertilization

*In vitro* just means 'in glass' and refers to a procedure in which living eggs are taken from a woman's ovary, fertilized by sperm in a sterile glass dish, and replaced in the uterus. There are no end of difficulties and the success rate is not high – no more than 10%. Ovulation is stimulated with drugs or hormones and the growth of the Graafian follicles checked by ultrasound. When a follicle reaches a size of about 1.5 mm, a dose of follicle-stimulating hormone is given to prompt the release of eggs. These, usually up to 10, are collected using a fine needle guided by the ultrasound image. The eggs are kept at body temperature in a suitable culture medium for four to six hours and then the sperm are added. The fertilized eggs are kept in the medium for about two days, and then two or three of them are placed in the uterus through a fine tube. Spare embryos can be frozen and kept for a later attempt if the first is not successful.

At present, in spite of remarkable advances, in vitro fertilization is the least successful way of dealing with infertility. In addition to the low success rate, babies born in this way have a somewhat higher chance of problems such as prematurity and developmental abnormalities. Tragically, as many as 50% of pregnancies brought about in this way do not result in an uncomplicated live birth. You should really consider it a last resort.

Gamete intrafallopian transfer (GIFT) is a method in which eggs are collected as described and then injected, along with some sperm, into the open end of one of the fallopian tubes. This is done through a laparoscope (see PELVIC EXAMINATION). This method is often effective in cases of unexplained infertility.

## Infibulation

See CIRCUMCISION OF WOMEN.

## Irritable bowel syndrome

This is the current term for a condition that has been known to doctors for many years under various names such as *spastic colon*, *nervous diarrhoea* or *idiopathic diarrhoea*. It is a persistent disorder for which no organic cause can be found. It features recurrent abdominal pain and intermittent diarrhoea often alternating with constipation.

This distressing disorder most commonly affects women between 20 and 40. The pain is usually felt in one of the four corners of the abdomen, is sometimes brought on by eating, and is often relieved by going to the toilet. The stools are usually ribbon-like or pellet-like and may contain mucus. Often, soon after a meal, there is extreme and embarrassing urgency to empty the bowels. There may be loud abdominal rumblings and squeaking (*borborygmi*), excessive gas production (*flatus*), headache, tiredness and nausea. Sometimes there is a sense of incomplete emptying after defaecation.

The condition tends to affect anxious, tense, intelligent, conscientious women, especially those who worry unduly about personal, family and financial matters. There may be an underlying fear of cancer. Full investigation, including barium meal X-ray, shows no objective abnormality, but, on examination, the colon is seen to be in a state of unusual activity, contracting and relaxing in an abnormally rapid manner.

A diet high in roughage is helpful in regulating the bowel action, and there are several drugs effective in quieting down the excessive bowel activity and relieving the pain. Drugs can be carried and taken in anticipation of events which might provoke an acute attack.

# K

## Kleptomania

This is a rare condition in which the sufferer repeatedly fails to resist the impulse to steal things she doesn't need or particularly want. The objects are usually taken from a shop. Kleptomaniacs are usually well able to pay for the things they steal and the motive is not the same as that of the thief.

The act is not usually pre-planned and the object is the theft itself rather than the acquisition. As in other impulse disorders, there is a rising sense of tension focused on the actual shoplifting, with a relief of tension and a sense of elation when the act is accomplished. This may, however, be followed by strong guilt feelings and intense fear of discovery. The stolen objects are usually given away or otherwise disposed of.

Although kleptomania is often put forward as a defence against a charge of theft, it is in fact very uncommon. Less than 5% of people arrested for shoplifting are found to respond to questioning in a manner consistent with the diagnosis of kleptomania. The condition is associated with stress, such as bereavement or separation, and kleptomaniacs also tend to suffer from persistent depression and ANOREXIA NERVOSA. Kleptomaniacs often seem to have given no thought to the probable consequences of their actions and some appear outraged if they are arrested. They have been described as people who feel wronged and thus entitled to steal.

The cause is unknown, but some very odd explanations have been proposed by psychoanalysts. These include the suggestion that:

## KLEPTOMANIA

- all stealing is rooted in the essential oneness between mother and child (Anna Freud)
- it represents a search for a penis
- it is a means of seeking punishment
- it is an excitement, enjoyed as a substitute for sexual intercourse

# L

## Labia

The labia (singular *labium*) are the four elongated lips that surround the entrance to your VAGINA and the external opening of the urine tube (*urethra*). The inner of the two pairs, the *labia minora*, are narrow, wrinkled and red and vary in depth in different women. Each one forks, at the front, to form a hood over the front of the head of the clitoris. The outer pair, the *labia majora*, are long, well padded folds, containing muscle and fatty tissue, and are covered with hair. At the front, they join in the lower part of the pubic mound (*mons veneris*). As they run back between the thighs, they become more prominent. Behind, they join together a few centimetres in front of the anus. They are normally closed and conceal the rest of the genitalia.

There is not much to go wrong with the labia apart from inflammation from THRUSH (*vulvitis*) or HERPES, genital warts or the effects of SEXUALLY TRANSMITTED DISEASES. Occasionally a large lip may be affected by an abscess in one of the BARTHOLIN'S GLANDS.

## Labour
See CHILDBIRTH.

## Laparoscopy
See PELVIC EXAMINATION.

## Lumpectomy

An operation for breast cancer in which no attempt is made to remove more than the obvious lump. Supplementary treatment with radiation or chemotherapy is then given. Lumpectomy is also used for benign lumps. See BREAST REMOVAL.

## Lymphoedema

This means persistent swelling of the tissues from blockage or absence of the lymph drainage vessels which carry tissue fluid (*lymph*) from the tissues back into the bloodstream. This may be caused by:

- deficiency of the lymph channels from birth, in which case it usually affects the legs
- operative removal, as in the surgical treatment of cancer
- obstruction by cancer cells
- obstruction by microscopic parasitic worms

The latter is a tropical disorder and causes elephantiasis.

Lymphoedema of the arm following surgical treatment or radiotherapy for cancer of the breast is difficult to treat. Success has been achieved, however, by tight compression with an elastic arm stocking and regular firm massage from the wrist to the armpit. It may be necessary to sleep with the arm raised in a sling above the level of the heart.

# M

## Mammography

Mammography is X-ray examination used in cases of suspected breast cancer and as a screening procedure for women. The value of mammography is still debated by some, but improvements in instruments and technique have increased its reliability, and most doctors now acknowledge its value. The procedure cannot be relied on to exclude cancer and does not distinguish between benign and malignant tumours. It does, however, often bring to light cases in which sampling of tissue (*biopsy*) is needed and, in this way, can lead to early diagnosis and cure of cancer.

About 40% of lumps cannot be felt, even by careful palpation, but may be detected by mammography. Of these, 20–30% contain cancer. Cysts, which are non-malignant, are easily visualized. Mammography is of little value to women under 35, but regular mammography is widely recommended for women over 50. The radiation dosage is very low and offers no significant risk.

The procedure, and position of the patient, varies with the type of machine, but is painless, although sometimes quite uncomfortable. A variety of methods is used to allow the soft tissue to be X-rayed without interference from other structures. The breasts may be laid on top of a flat surface or allowed to hang down; they may be sucked into a cavity, or may be gently squeezed between plates.

## Mastectomy
See BREAST REMOVAL.

## Mastitis
See BREAST INFLAMMATION.

## ME
See MYALGIC ENCEPHALITIS.

## Menopause
The menopause or climacteric is the natural end of the sequence of menstrual periods and the end of the fertile years of life in a woman. The menopause occurs at an average age of about 50 but the usual range is from 48 to 54. Occurrences outside this range are quite common. A premature menopause occurs if the ovaries are removed surgically (*oophorectomy*). The menopause involves a cessation of egg production (*ovulation*) by the ovaries and of the resulting hormonal changes which alter the inner lining of the UTERUS.

The main effect of the menopause is a reduced production of the hormone oestrogen by the ovaries. Some of the symptoms and effects of the menopause are due to oestrogen deficiency, but, for some women, the awareness that they have come to the end of reproductive life and have reached a significant stage in ageing, may have as much effect as the hormone deficiency. The menopause often coincides with the departure of the last of the now grown-up children from the family home, and a mother may suffer the feeling that she is now less valued.

Most women pass easily through the menopause and are relatively unaffected. Many are relieved to be spared the risk of pregnancy or the need for contraception. About a quarter suffer in some way, mainly from hot flushes, night sweats, insomnia, headaches and general irritability. Often these symptoms are severe enough, in themselves, to justify treatment. It is by no means certain that these symptoms are due to oestrogen deficiency – this has never been proved. But the placebo effect of oestrogen treatment is strong and most women and their doctors believe it responsible for the resulting improvement.

A lack of oestrogen causes thinning of the wall of the VAGINA and a reduction in lubricating secretions in about a quarter of postmenopausal women. This can cause difficulty and discomfort in sexual intercourse but is easily corrected by HORMONE REPLACEMENT THERAPY (HRT), either with an oestrogen alone or with combined oestrogen and progesterone treatment. For long-term use, the latter is safer but has the disadvantage that menstrual bleeding continues. The important sign of postmenopausal bleeding – a possible indication of cancer – may be obscured.

Oestrogens are strongly protective against the major arterial and heart diseases in non-smoking women, and this protection is lost after the menopause. This is held by many to be an added justification for hormone replacement therapy. Loss of bone bulk and OSTEOPOROSIS is a natural feature of ageing, but reduced oestrogen accelerates the process in postmenopausal women. This is a strong indication for hormone replacement therapy.

Contrary to widespread belief, the menopause is not associated with a marked increase in psychiatric disturbance. Most women find, to their surprise, that conventional Western attitudes and beliefs about the menopause are exaggerated and unnecessarily alarmist. But they are part of the cultural tradition and continue to be perpetuated in spite of much evidence to the contrary.

## Menorrhagia
Excessive bleeding during a menstrual period. See PERIOD PROBLEMS.

## Menstrual problems
See PERIOD PROBLEMS.

## Miscarriage
It is believed that as many as one in five pregnancies end in spontaneous miscarriage. Miscarriage may be caused by abnormal chromosomes so that a fetus, which would have grown to be an abnormal baby, is discarded. The developing fetus may implant at an unsuitable site in the uterus; the uterus may be abnormal or the neck of the uterus (*cervix*) too weak to retain the growing fetus. The mother may be producing insufficient hormones (especially progesterone) to maintain the pregnancy or there may be infection of the reproductive organs. All these can lead to miscarriage. In most cases the cause of spontaneous abortion is not identified.

The unmistakable sign of *threatened abortion* is bleeding, or a dark brown discharge, from the VAGINA. Often there is a slight pain, like a period pain, in the lower abdomen. Although the embryo or fetus remains alive and still attached to the wall of the uterus, the bleeding indicates that there is a threat of separation. About a quarter of these will go on to miscarriage, but most settle down, and the pregnancy continues to full term with delivery of a healthy, normal baby. In such cases, threatened abortion does not imply that there is anything wrong with the baby.

If the bleeding gets worse and the pain becomes more severe and cramping, there comes a point when it has to be recognized that miscarriage is inevitable. Inevitable abortion means that the cervix has opened and the contents of the uterus are being expelled by contractions. Blood clots and membranes, enclosing the fetus, will have passed into the VAGINA. Sometimes bleeding from an inevitable abortion is so severe as to call for a blood transfusion.

Often the expulsion is incomplete and a minor operation, under general anaesthesia, may be needed. This is called evacuation of retained products of conception (ERPC). The uterus is emptied by suction and the lining is carefully scraped with a sharp-edged spoon called a curette. A drug is then given to cause the uterus to contract and antibiotics may also be necessary. The patient is usually able to go home the next day.

Sometimes the fetus dies but is retained in the uterus. This is called *missed abortion*. In this case there is often a history of threatened miscarriage that has apparently settled. But later, the signs of pregnancy – morning sickness, breast enlargement and tenderness – disappear. A brownish discharge may occur. Suspicion that this has happened can be confirmed by ULTRA-SOUND SCANNING, which will no longer show a fetal heart beat. In the end the remaining material is usually expelled spontaneously, but an ERPC is often necessary.

Most miscarriages occur in the early weeks of pregnancy. Later miscarriage is less common and may mean that there is something wrong with the uterus or that the cervix is unable to remain closed. This is described by doctors as CERVICAL INCOMPETENCE. In the latter case, the cervix opens up, with little or no pain and minimal bleeding and the baby is lost. This can usually be prevented in subsequent pregnancies by the use of a string tied around the neck of the uterus to strengthen the cervix. This is called a cervical suture.

Some women abort repeatedly and are described as 'habitual aborters'. Gynaecological investigation will reveal the cause in about 40% of cases.

## Morning sickness
See PREGNANCY COMPLICATIONS.

## Myalgic encephalitis
*Encephalitis* means 'inflammation of the brain' and *myalgic* means 'relating to muscle pain'. The concept of myalgic encephalitis (ME) has been the cause of much silent suffering in women. It has also deeply divided the medical profession for years and has provoked sometimes acrimonious and dismissive argument between those who believe the condition entirely imaginary and those who think it has an organic basis. The often derogatory remarks made about people with this problem and the implication that most of them are malingerers or manipulators betrays the common but somewhat outdated notion that the mind and the body are entirely separable.

There is no questioning the existence of a common and serious disorder, affecting predominantly women, that features severe fatigue and emotional disturbance. The condition is made worse by exercise, a single act of which may cause fatigue for weeks. Unfortunately, these effects have been variously associated with a great number of other symptoms and signs, and a range of names has been applied to what may or may not be the same condition. These names include the Royal Free disease, epidemic neuromyasthenia, Otago mystery disease, Icelandic disease, institutional mass hysteria, benign myalgic encephalomyelitis and the postviral fatigue syndrome.

The basic difficulty, so far as medical attitudes are concerned, stems from two points; firstly, medical awareness that complaint of persistent fatigue is often a feature of neurotic illness in which the sufferer is seeking a resolution of some major personal or social problem; and secondly, the failure of medical investigation to find a cause.

Virus infection has been widely proposed as a cause of the syndrome and a wide range of viruses including Coxsackie, herpes, polio, varicella-zoster (chickenpox and shingles) and Epstein-Barr (glandular fever) have been cited. Unfortunately, the finding of antibodies to these or other viruses in people with ME proves nothing. The world is full of people with such antibodies who do not have ME. Moreover, psychological stress increases susceptibility to infection, so even a higher than normal prevalence of these antibodies in ME sufferers would not prove that viruses are the cause. Extensive immunological studies into people with ME have been inconclusive.

Although the condition is called an encephalitis, none of the normal neurological tests, such as electroencephalography, show that this is present. Some tests on muscle fibres have shown abnormalities in some cases but these have not been universally accepted.

It is clear that the 'fatigue' experienced by ME sufferers is not a matter of the muscles alone and is quite different from the weakness experienced in muscular disorders such as myasthenia gravis. The fatigue of ME has a strong cognitive element and is commonly associated with mild to severe depression. A comparison of the bodily effects of depression – fatigue, headache, breathlessness, chest pain, dizziness and often bowel upset – with those of ME shows a striking similarity. The prevalences of ME and of depression are also very similar. In some cases the syndrome has responded well to treatment with antidepressant drugs.

Derogatory attitudes on the part of doctors and others have not been helpful and have caused great distress to sufferers who have often been forced to turn to alternative therapists. Whether the condition is of external organic origin or otherwise is, currently, the central point at issue. But it is equally important to acknowledge that people whose lives are as severely affected as those of ME sufferers, deserve as much help as any similarly affected people, whatever the cause. Such a gross and persistent disruption of normal living indicates a major disorder of the whole person and can, in no sense, be considered to be 'all in the mind'.

## Myxoedema

A term used to describe the general effects of severe underactivity of the thyroid gland. This occurs in women five times as often as in men. The skin is dry and scaly, cold, thickened and coarse. The hair is scanty, coarse and brittle. Often the eyebrows are greatly thinned or even partly absent. The lips are thickened and mauve-coloured and there is halitosis. The affected person does not complain, but is lethargic, readily fatigued, slowed in body and mind and suffers muscle aches, loss of menstruation, deafness, angina pectoris, heart failure, ANAEMIA and constipation.

All these effects can be reversed by the administration of thyroid hormones.

# N

## Nail disorders

Because of their position, and the constant use of the hands, fingernails are vulnerable to injury. Commonly, as a result of injury, a collection of blood (*haematoma*) forms under the nail, and this may affect nail adhesion. Detachment of the nail from its bed is called *onycholysis*. Apart from injury, onycholysis may be caused by psoriasis, fungus infection and thyroid gland overactivity. The separation usually starts at the tip and extends backwards. Air under the nail gives it a greyish-white colour. A complete, spontaneous shedding of one or more nails can occur in any severe illness as this can lead to a sudden cessation of nail growth and lack of adhesion of the plate to the bed. Toenails are also susceptible to injury, often repeated, and this may lead to a condition of very marked thickening, and claw-like curving, known as *onychogryphosis*.

*Paronychia*, the infection of the soft tissue around the nail, is probably the commonest of all nail disorders. It most commonly affects the toes and is popularly, but incorrectly, known as 'ingrowing toenail'. There is pain, swelling and inflammation, and sometimes pus appears at the nail edge. The condition usually results from repeated minor injury and working conditions which make proper hand care difficult. Fungus infection of the nails (*onychomycosis*) is common and causes thickening, distortion and separation. It is hard to treat but will respond to the drug griseofulvin which must be taken for at least a year. Unfortunately there may be side effects.

Small point-like depressions (pits) occur in the persistent skin disease psoriasis and in patchy baldness (*alopecia areata*). Single horizontal ridges that move along, with growth, towards the tip of the nail may indicate a previous illness. Multiple horizontal ridges suggest infection in the skin around the nail bed. Longitudinal ridges occur in alopecia areata, psoriasis and in the very itchy skin disease lichen planus. Nail thickening is common in psoriasis and fungus infection. The small white patches occurring on most people's nails have never been adequately explained.

## Natural childbirth

This term was used by pioneers of prepared, or educated childbirth, such as Dr Grantly Dick-Read, Margaret Gamper and Elizabeth Bing, to try to attract women to the concept that giving birth is, or should be, a normal and natural process rather than a kind of medical or surgical disorder. The work of these pioneers has proved invaluable to countless millions of women who have found that a clear and full understanding of what to expect, and instruction in relaxation and cooperation, can make labour much less difficult and painful and more rewarding. The preparation is primarily psychological and is based, in part, on an understanding of the nature of pain and of how this is influenced by the state of mind and the condition of tension in the muscles. Women are shown how fear and ignorance breed muscle tension and a state of mind in which the perception of pain, and sensitivity to it, are much higher than necessary.

The natural childbirth movement is now part of the routine of childbirth and is available to almost all women who want it. If you are in your first pregnancy you are strongly advised to attend classes.

## Nipple disorders

The nipple is the central prominence of each breast, larger in women than in men. The word derives from the Anglo-Saxon *nib*, meaning 'a little beak'. In women, 15 to 20 milk ducts pass from the milk-producing lobes of the breast out through each nipple. The area surrounding the nipple is called the areola and this is a pinkish colour in those who have not been pregnant, but darker in those who have. Erection of the nipple occurs in the cold, on light touch, on sexual excitement and on the stimulus of breast feeding.

Nipples are sometimes naturally turned inwards (*inverted*) and this can cause feeding problems. Inverted nipples should be regularly pulled out. A naturally inverted nipple should be distinguished from a previously normal nipple which becomes indrawn or distorted. This may be a sign of cancer and should be reported to a doctor at once.

Cracked and sore nipples are common features of breast-feeding. Cracked nipples can allow access to infective organisms and may lead to a BREAST ABSCESS. Cracks should be allowed to heal even if breastfeeding must be stopped for a day or two and the milk expressed and given from a bottle. Sore nipples sometimes occur when the nipple is pulled from the baby's mouth instead of breaking the suction with a finger. Teething babies should be firmly stopped from biting. Sore nipples should be exposed as much as possible and allowed to dry after feeds. See also BREASTFEEDING and PAGET'S DISEASE OF THE NIPPLE.

## Nose shaping

Rhinoplasty is an operation to alter the structure of the nose for cosmetic reasons. This is done either to correct a deformity caused by injury or disease or to improve the appearance of a healthy nose.

The surgery is performed within the nose to avoid visible scarring. Under a general anaesthetic, incisions are made in the inner lining – the mucous membrane – to uncover the wall of cartilage and bone that divides the nose into two cavities (*nasal septum*). The surgeon then works between the skin and the cartilage to reshape it, using a fine scalpel and forceps. Any surplus bone is removed with a chisel or a rasp. If necessary, the nose can be built up with bone grafts taken from another part of the body. The new shape of the nose is retained with a plaster mould for about ten days.

# O

## Obesity

See WEIGHT PROBLEMS.

## Osteoporosis

Our bones are made mainly of a tough, elastic protein called collagen organized along efficient engineering lines to produce maximum strength with minimum weight. But bones made solely of collagen would be rubbery and useless so the entire collagen structure is reinforced and stiffened with calcium and phosphorus. If, for any reason, there is a shortage of minerals, especially calcium, the reinforcement becomes inadequate and bones will soften and may bend under the body weight. This occurs in rickets in children and osteomalacia in adults, usually because calcium is not being absorbed properly from the intestine because of a deficiency of vitamin D. In osteoporosis, however, the basic problem is not a deficiency of minerals.

Like the rest of the tissues of your body, living bones are in a state of constant physical and chemical change, losing and gaining dissolved calcium, phosphorus and the protein subunits, the amino acids, to and from your bloodstream. The movement of these substances is controlled by various growth and sex hormones some of which reduce, and some of which increase, the amounts that are deposited in your bones. Changes in the amounts of these hormones can thus greatly affect the strength of your bones, both in mineral and in protein terms.

## The sex hormones and the bones

The most important hormones in this respect are the sex hormones. You probably think of the sex hormones as substances that determine gender and sexuality. This is true, but an equally important effect of the sex hormones is to make people stronger. Sex hormones, both male and female, are steroids and they are *anabolic*. The word simply means 'building up'. The sudden growth spurt at puberty and the physical changes in the body are due to sex hormones. Male sex hormones are more anabolic than female. This gives men a double advantage over women in relation to bone strength – first, because of the greater anabolic effect and second, because men go on producing their sex hormones throughout life while women stop producing them at the time of the menopause. Because of this, and because men start off with thicker bones than women, osteoporosis is essentially a woman's problem. Soon after the menopause the loss of density in women's bones tends to accelerate and in 20 years the loss can be considerable and dangerous.

Other hormones, and also hormone drugs, can affect bone strength. One of the hormones from the adrenal glands is called cortisol. This is a *catabolic* ('breaking-down') steroid and too much cortisol or other corticosteroids can be very bad for the bones and may rapidly cause osteoporosis. In the disease known as Cushing's syndrome, overproduction of cortisol by one or both adrenal glands causes osteoporosis. There is a large range of corticosteroid drugs which are identical to, or closely similar to, cortisol. These steroids also cause osteoporosis and this danger should be balanced against their importance in the management of other conditions. For this and other reasons the steroids should never be used without good reason.

In addition to the steroids, various natural body hormones control the amounts of calcium and phosphorus in the bones. Disorders of these hormone glands can lead to softening or undue hardening of the bones, as minerals are leached out or over-deposited.

## Strength from use

There is another important factor that can influence the strength of your bones. Bones are thickest and strongest in early adult life, thereafter becoming gradually thinner with age as a result of progressive loss of the protein structure and of minerals. This occurs for an unexpected reason. The rate of decline in bone strength is affected to an important degree by the demands we make on them. Bones stay strong by being used and by having physical forces, such as those involved in weight-bearing, walking, running and so on, applied to them. These physical forces actually stimulate the bone-forming cells into action so that the need for greater strength is met. This is an example of the many ways in which the body reacts to external demand.

Under-use of the bones, as occurs in bed-ridden people or in astronauts living in zero gravity, leads to osteoporosis. Even a change from an active to a sedentary life as a result of arthritis or some other disabling condition, will cause osteoporosis. And, of course, the ordinary processes of ageing, with associated loss of activity and reduced hormone levels, will inevitably cause it. Women should be especially aware of the importance of keeping up the levels of activity throughout life.

### The effects of osteoporosis

These are as common as they are severe. A quarter of a million thighbone neck fractures occur in the USA, and nearly 40 000 in Britain, every year. Four-fifths of these are attributable, wholly or partially, to osteoporosis. The cost of treating osteoporosis-related medical conditions in the USA is about six billion dollars a year. Unfortunately, osteoporosis causes no symptoms until some effect of the weakening in the bones occurs. The commonest effect of all is an unexpected fracture of the neck of the hip bone as a result of a quite minor stumble or fall. Thirty per cent of women over the age of 60 suffer this misfortune and the consequences are often very serious. In spite of brilliant improvements in the orthopaedic surgical management of fracture of the neck of the femur, this disaster still commonly shortens life. Twenty-five per cent of women over 60 suffer fractures of the spinal bones (*vertebrae*) as a result of osteoporosis. The extent of the problem is partly concealed by uncomplaining, patient women who attribute their symptoms to 'old age' and do not seek medical help.

Other effects of osteoporosis include:

- fracture of the wrist from minor stress
- persistent severe back pain
- loss of height from shrinkage of the bones of the spinal column
- sudden collapse of one of the bones of the spine with severe pain and 'dowager's hump' disfigurement
- severe and progressive curvature of the spine so that the body becomes ever more bent

Such osteoporotic spinal curvature (*kyphosis*) is disfiguring and, especially if there was a previous tendency to stooping, may sometimes become so extreme as to force the chin on to the chest and even interfere with eating. Many women become so embarrassed over their appearance that they go out as little as possible, avoid social contacts and become reclusive.

### Kyphosis

An abnormal degree of backward curvature of part of the spine is called kyphosis. The term comes from the Greek *kyphos* meaning 'bowed or bent', and is used to describe a degree of backward curvature of the spine sufficient to cause deformity.

Kyphosis is due to downward loading on the spine so that the normal curves are exaggerated. This will not happen unless there is inadequate support, either from poor muscles, faulty posture or weakening of the bones. It therefore tends to affect two groups – adolescents, as a result of slouching or slumping and postmenopausal women as a result of osteo-porosis. Progressive kyphosis from osteoporosis calls for ener-getic medical management. Neglected, the outcome may be one of serious height loss, gross deformity and sometimes major disability.

### What should you do about it?

Once osteoporosis has developed it is very difficult to restore bone strength. So there are many good reasons to try to mini-mize the rate of loss of bone bulk. Taking regular exercise, as strenuous as is reasonable and safe, is one obvious measure you should never neglect. Taking plenty of calcium – at least

1,500 mg per day – is harmless and distinctly worthwhile. For some inexplicable reason, cigarette smoking is associated with increased osteoporosis. This is just one of the many strong reasons why smoking should be avoided. Moderation in alcohol intake is also recommended for this and other reasons.

There is now complete medical agreement that oestrogen HORMONE REPLACEMENT THERAPY (HRT) significantly reduces the risk of osteoporosis in women after the menopause. Oestrogens unquestionably retard the process of loss of bone substance, but do not lead to an increase in bone bulk. Unfortunately, they do have some disadvantages, especially in producing a slight increase in the risk of breast and UTERUS cancer. In spite of this, most doctors are strongly in favour of oestrogen HRT. There is good evidence that calcium supplements in the diet also help. A recent large multinational study of the effects of oestrogens, calcium and calcitonin on women over 50 reported in the *British Medical Journal* in November, 1992, showed that all three supplements significantly reduced the risk of hip fracture.

The decision is, of course, yours, but it should be an informed decision. If you are in a category with a slight increase in the risk of breast cancer – perhaps because your mother has or had this misfortune – you may feel that the slightly increased risk should not be taken. At the same time, it is important for you to know that the mortality rate from breast cancer (as well as from other causes) is significantly lower in women on HRT than in comparable groups not taking it. If you already know, from X-ray or other scanning evidence, that you have a degree of osteoporosis and if you are a naturally small-boned person, you owe it to yourself to consider seriously what you should do to minimize the risks of future bone problems. HRT by the skin patch method is more effective and has fewer side effects than HRT by mouth. The risk of uterus cancer can be eliminated by adding progesterone to the oestrogen.

## Ovarian cancer

Cancer of the ovary is commoner in women who have never had children than in those who have. It may occur at any age but is most usual between 50 and 60. Unfortunately, ovarian cancer tends to be symptomless ('silent') until it has grown and spread, displacing and invading the UTERUS and spreading widely within the pelvis and abdomen. Diagnosis is usually made by direct viewing with a fine instrument called an endoscope, which is passed through the wall of the abdomen.

The treatment is surgical and the uterus and both ovaries must be removed as the second ovary often also contains a tumour. Ovarian cancer is often very susceptible to anti-cancer chemotherapy. Radiotherapy is seldom useful.

## Ovarian cysts

These can occur at any age, but are commonest between 35 and 55. Most of them produce no symptoms and the only sign is a gradual increase in the size of the abdomen which is often attributed to simple obesity. Ovarian cysts can become very large, however, and may press on and partially obstruct the large pelvic veins leading to varicose veins or piles (*haemorrhoids*). They can also compress the urine tubes from the kidneys (*ureters*) and cause kidney damage. Their sheer bulk can cause breathlessness and abdominal discomfort. Women sometimes mistake this enlargement for a pregnancy.

Cysts may be caused by slight disorders of ovulation or by distention of the delicate outer lining of the ovary from fluid collection. Such swellings are usually harmless. Cysts caused in this way usually pass unnoticed, but occasionally they grow big enough to cause pain. Treatment is seldom required.

The commonest true ovarian cysts are called serous cysts and contain watery fluid. These occur late in the reproductive life or after the menopause and may be of almost any size up to an enormous bulk, filling and distending the abdomen. The similar pseudomucinous cysts contain a viscous mucoid fluid and may also grow very large. These cysts cause trouble mainly by their bulk, but may cause severe complications if they become twisted and their blood supply is cut off or if they rupture or become infected. Surgeons are very careful to avoid damaging the capsule when removing pseudomucinous cysts, as the contents are very irritating to the inner lining of the abdomen (*peritoneum*), and cells can be released which can set up new cysts elsewhere in the abdomen. Ovarian cysts may result from ENDOMETRIOSIS of the ovary. These contain altered blood and almost always cause pain. Surgical treatment is usually necessary.

## Ovaries

These are the basic female gonads of central importance to your sexual development. Your ovaries are situated in your pelvis, one on each side of the UTERUS, just under, and inward of, the open ends of the FALLOPIAN TUBES. Your ovaries are almond-shaped and about 3 cm long, with prominent blood vessels. Each ovary contains many ovum sites known as

*Graafian follicles*. Once a month, one of these, or sometimes more than one, matures, swells up a little, ruptures and releases an ovum. This is called ovulation. Ovulation sometimes causes minor pain known as 'middle pain' or *mittelschmerz*. After ovulation, each ruptured follicle is replaced by a yellow body known as a *corpus luteum*. In addition to producing ova, your ovaries synthesize three types of steroid hormone – oestrogens, progesterones (both of which are female sex hormones) and androgens, which, believe it or not, are male sex hormones. The male sex hormones are anabolic and are quite useful in helping you to develop good muscles. Fortunately, they are not normally able to overcome the feminizing effect of the female sex hormones.

## Ovum

The egg, or ovum, is the female reproductive cell (*gamete*), produced by one or other of your ovaries about halfway between two menstrual periods. Your ovaries usually produce one egg per month, but may produce more than one. The egg contains 23 of the 46 chromosomes needed to make a new individual. The other 23 are supplied by the sperm at the moment of fertilization. The egg is a very large cell, as cells go, much larger than a sperm, and is about 0.1 mm in diameter. This is by far the largest cell in your body. Like all eggs it is large because it has to contain food (*yolk*) to keep the embryo nourished during its earliest stages before it can establish a supply from the mother via the placenta.

If more than one egg is produced and fertilized, a multiple pregnancy results, but the babies are not identical because, in each case, half the chromosomes come from different sperms, with different genetic material. But if a fertilized ovum divides and each of the two halves forms a new individual, these will be identical twins, with identical chromosomes.

At birth the ovaries contain about a million immature ova. Only about four hundred of these immature ova become mature and are released. No new ova are produced after birth and all those that may be fertilized are the same age as the woman. This is why there is a slight tendency for genetic abnormalities to be commoner in babies born to older women. The ova have had longer to develop mutations.

# P

## Paget's disease of the nipple

It is quite common for an itchy skin rash to affect both breasts. This is often a form of eczema, calling for treatment with ointments. But if a patch of reddened skin, resembling eczema, appears on only one nipple, it is possible that, under it, is a small cancer. This may be so even if you cannot feel a lump. This is called Paget's disease of the nipple.

Such a patch should always be reported. Usually a biopsy, to exclude or confirm cancer, is required. Paget's disease does not readily spread beyond the breast tissue, but should always be removed. Undue delay is dangerous. There is also a Paget's disease of bone, but this is quite a different condition.

## Partner counselling

Much discord between partners arises from difficulty, or refusal, to see matters from the other's point of view. Differences can sometimes be resolved if an agreed third person, who is able to take a detached and unbiased view, is brought into the situation. Communication between partners can be re-established and damaging behaviour patterns, that are obvious to an outside observer but not apparent to the participants, can be pointed out and examined.

Ideally, partner counselling calls for an experienced, wise and unprejudiced counsellor – a person who can gain the respect of, and whose advice can be accepted by, even the most apparently unreasonable. The difficulty is to find such a paragon. No special school of psychology has a monopoly on counselling, but the ideas and methods of the behaviourists – which are largely based on common sense – seem to be more effective than most. Essentially sexual problems, although often important in causing discord, are not primarily the concern of counsellors. In cases where such problems are central, the couple may be referred to an appropriate expert.

To a large extent, success in counselling is dependent on a genuine desire for reconciliation and on the importance each partner places on the relationship. Often, unfortunately, it is much more important to one than to the other.

## Pelvic examination

This is often called 'vaginal examination', but the gynaecologist is not so much concerned with the VAGINA as with what may be felt in the pelvis by way of the vagina. This examination involves both hands, the second being used to feel through the front wall of your abdomen. Pelvic examination is often quite uncomfortable, and if there are any inflamed parts within your pelvis, pressure on them will cause pain. The doctor wants to know about this, so being brave is not particularly helpful. The important thing, however, is to try to relax everything as much as you can. This will make it easier for you and the doctor.

Direct visual examination of the interior of the pelvis is called laparoscopy. This is done using fibreoptic illumination and viewing channels contained in a narrow viewing tube (*endoscope*), which can be passed through a small cut in the wall of your abdomen. Laparoscopy can be used by any specialist concerned with disease of the abdominal organs, but has been especially adopted by gynaecologists for the investigation of disorders of the female reproductive organs in the pelvis. Conditions, such as ectopic pregnancy, and sterility from possible obstruction of the fallopian tubes, which are difficult to diagnose with certainty in any other way short of an exploratory abdominal operation, can be diagnosed in this way. Laparoscopy also allows a range of operations to be performed and is widely used as a means of deliberately closing off the fallopian tubes to achieve sterilization. Laparoscopy can be valuable in the diagnosis of doubtful cases of appendicitis, or diseases of the gall bladder or liver.

Laparoscopy is usually done under general anaesthesia. Harmless carbon dioxide gas is passed in through a small needle to inflate the abdominal cavity and move the intestines out of the way. The endoscope can then be safely inserted through a small incision. Various instruments, including laser channels, can be passed through the laparoscope, for diverse purposes. In particular, tissues can be vaporized and cut, without bleeding; local disease, such as patches of ENDOMETRIOSIS, destroyed; and biopsies can be taken from any organ, including the liver. Eggs (*ova*) can be taken from the ovaries for *in vitro fertilization* (see INFERTILITY). The pressure of the gas in the abdomen may cause some discomfort for a day or two, until it absorbs. There may also be referred pain from irritation of the diaphragm. This is felt in the tip of the shoulder.

In videolaseroscopy or videoendoscopy, a video camera is attached to the laparoscope so that the interior of the abdomen can be viewed on a TV monitor and the procedure carried out while watching the screen. This is convenient for the surgeon who, in the past, has had to spend long periods bending over the patient's abdomen looking through a single small eye-piece. Zoom magnification of small areas is possible and videotape recordings can be made.

## Pelvic measurement

This is called pelvimetry and it is sometimes done to assess the area of the outlet of the female pelvis so as to anticipate difficulty in delivery of the baby. A rough assessment can be made by checking the distance between the prominent bones behind the buttocks (*ischial tuberosities*) on vaginal examination. More precise measurements can be made by various X-ray techniques, but the use of X-rays in this region is avoided, if possible, during pregnancy, and the method is seldom used nowadays.

Even so, radiological pelvimetry may occasionally be justified in women with a history of difficult or prolonged labour, when safer methods of imaging are not available. It may even be needed for women already in labour if the fetal head has failed to engage, or in breech presentation with a large baby. The later in pregnancy, the lower the radiation risk to the fetus.

## Pelvis

The pelvis is the bony girdle formed by the two hip bones on either side and the triangular curved sacrum, behind. The hip bones are held together in front by a midline joint called the pubic symphysis. Behind, each hip bone is attached to the sacrum at one of the two sacroiliac joints. Each hip bone contains a deep, spherical cup, called the acetabulum, into which the head of the thigh bone (*femur*) fits.

The sacroiliac joints are the semi-rigid ligamentous junctions, at the back, holding the two outer bones of the pelvis to the side surfaces of the sacrum. The coccyx, or tail bone, consists of four small vertebrae fused together and joined to the curved sacrum. Normally very little movement occurs at the sacroiliac joints, but late in pregnancy the strong ligaments holding the joints together become more lax, so as to allow easier childbirth. The width of your hips depends on the width of your pelvis and on the angle with which the heads of your two thigh bones articulate with it.

Experts can easily distinguish a female pelvis from a male, by its proportions. The female pelvis is relatively wider and shallower than the male and the lower opening (the outlet) is better shaped to allow a baby's head to pass. The lower part of the sacrum is also more flexible in the female.

## Period problems

Since menstruation is the result of hormonal influences on a structure which is, itself, liable to a variety of diseases, the range of menstrual disorders is considerable.

### Premenstrual tension (PMT)

This is a state of heightened mental tension with various physical symptoms that affects some women between the time of ovulation and the start of the next period. The symptoms improve as soon as the period has started and usually pass altogether until about ten days before the next period. It mainly affects women over 30. Symptoms of PMT include:

- a general feeling of illness (*malaise*)
- irritability or anger

- depression
- loss of concentration
- loss of energy
- insomnia or over-sleeping
- backache
- discomfort in the pelvis
- a sense of bloating
- headache
- soreness of the breasts
- weight gain of up to 1 kg

The weight gain is due to fluid and salt retention. Medical opinion is divided on the reality or significance of PMT but many women will testify that they suffer badly at this time. PMT has been accepted as a legal defence on the grounds of diminished responsibility, but this fact is of no medical significance. Some doctors think that PMT is due to a relative over-production of oestrogen, compared with progesterone, in the second half of the cycle.

Maybe you can persuade your doctor to prescribe a drug to encourage urination (a *diuretic* such as chlorothiazide) so as to get rid of the surplus water. This can give you a lot of relief. Progesterone by injection or by mouth will also relieve premenstrual tension in many cases. A mild tranquillizer may be necessary.

### Painful menstruation
This is called dysmenorrhoea and is very common, having been experienced by almost all women from time to time. Just before, or at the beginning of the period, there is cramping, rhythmical pain in the lower abdomen and back, lasting usu-

ally for a few hours, but sometimes for a day, or even throughout the period. The pain is associated with strong contractions of the UTERUS and with opening (*dilatation*) of the neck of the uterus (*cervix*). There may also be nausea, vomiting, diarrhoea, and cramping, colicky pain in the bowels. Some women have faintness and dizziness. In about 10% it is severe enough to cause temporary disability.

Dysmenorrhoea is almost always cured by having a baby, but less drastic remedies can also be effective. Drugs of the antiprostaglandin type ((Brufen, Panadol and Aspirin) are useful, and in severe cases, menstruation can be stopped altogether by means of oral contraceptives, taken continuously. This should be done only under medical supervision.

The condition may also result as a secondary effect of pelvic infection and other local disease, such as uterine fibroids or ENDOMETRIOSIS and, in these cases, antibiotics for infection or surgery may be necessary to effect a cure.

### Absence of periods

Amenorrhoea is the absence of menstruation and this may be primary (in girls of menstrual age who have not started to menstruate) or secondary, in those who have already had periods. Primary amenorrhoea may be due to hormonal causes, stress, or an imperforate hymen which completely closes off the vaginal outlet. The commonest cause of secondary amenorrhoea is, of course, pregnancy, but after that amenorrhoea is probably most often caused by ANOREXIA NERVOSA or by severe nutritional inadequacy. Amenorrhoea also occurs in athletes engaged in sustained, very vigorous training. Oligomenorrhea means infrequent or scanty periods.

## Too much bleeding (*menorrhagia*)

Menorrhagia means excessive bleeding during periods occurring at normal intervals. Polymenorrhea means having periods more often than every three weeks. Metrorrhagia is bleeding between periods.

Heavy periods lasting for seven or eight days with frequent passage of clots are normal for some women and may continue throughout the menstrual life. But if your normal period is three to four days of light bleeding and bleeding such as this were to occur, this would represent menorrhagia. In any case, a period requiring a change of tampon or pad every hour, for more than a few hours, indicates an abnormality likely to require medical attention.

Menorrhagia is most commonly due to an excessive build-up of the endometrium – the inner lining of the UTERUS – and this is controlled by oestrogen. Progesterone, which comes from the follicle in the ovary after the ovum is released, controls the bleeding. At the beginning and the end of the menstrual life, periods often occur without ovulation, so in the absence of progesterone, the periods may be very heavy. Progesterone may be used to control this type of menorrhagia.

Another cause of heavy vaginal bleeding is spontaneous ABORTION and this often occurs without pregnancy being suspected. Up to 10% of pregnancies end in this way, and the retained products may cause heavy bleeding. In this case, the bleeding can be stopped by a DILATATION AND CURETTAGE (D and C).

Fibroid tumours and polyps may cause excessive bleeding, as may cancer of the endometrium of the uterus, but the latter is likely to cause irregular bleeding, rather than menorrhagia.

**Irregularity**

A misleading term used to describe the effect of a variety of influences, including the occasional missed periods that occur normally at the beginning of the menstrual life and at the time of the MENOPAUSE. A common cause of apparent irregularity is pregnancy followed by MISCARRIAGE at a very early stage. Often, pregnancy may be unsuspected.

Periods missed as a result of anorexia, excessive dieting, or strenuous athletics may also cause an apparent irregularity. Another common cause is midcycle bleeding, when, at the time of ovulation, oestrogen levels may briefly drop sufficiently to allow the uterus lining to break down.

The appearance of menstrual irregularity may result from abnormal bleeding from other causes. When there is inflammation of the VAGINA or cervix, bleeding may occur after intercourse. Bleeding may result from trauma to polyps or tumours. It may also be due to ENDOMETRIOSIS, to cancer of the endometrium or to the presence of an IUD (*intrauterine contraceptive device*).

**Pessary**

A pessary is a small medicated vaginal plug or suppository, usually containing a drug, an antiseptic or a spermicide. The active substance is dissolved in a waxy vehicle, such as coconut butter, that melts at body temperature. This is a convenient and effective way of applying medication to the VAGINA.

The term is also used to describe one of various devices, often ring-shaped, inserted in the vagina to correct downward displacement (*prolapse*) or retroversion of the uterus. Another type, the diaphragm pessary, is used as a barrier method of contraception.

## Phobias

These are intense, irrational fears which cannot be ignored or overcome even when the sufferer is fully aware, as is usually the case, that there is no reason for the fear. Phobias take many forms and include fear of humiliation or embarrassment (social phobias), fear of high places (*acrophobia*), fear of open places (*agoraphobia*), fear of spiders (*arachnophobia*), fear of enclosed places (*claustrophobia*), fear of cats (*gatophobia*), fear of water (*hydrophobia*), fear of dead bodies (*necrophobia*), fear of darkness (*nyctophobia*), fear of crowds (*ochlophobia*) and fear of animals (*zoophobia*).

Phobias may relate to almost any situation, idea or object and most people have at least one mild phobia. Severe phobias are, however, very disabling and can seriously disrupt normal living. Most people have a reasonable fear of cancer, but cancer phobia has nothing to do with reason. It is a distressing personality disorder of the *phobic* type, with the attention of the affected person directed towards cancer.

Cancer phobia, unfortunately, does not prompt the sufferer to rational courses such as regular breast screening, BREAST SELF-EXAMINATION, CERVICAL SMEAR TESTS (*Pap smears*), avoidance of risk factors such as smoking, and so on. Instead, it gives rise to compulsively performed rituals, especially repeated handwashing, changing of clothes that have been touched by others, avoidance of air breathed by others, and even avoidance of any contact with other people. Symptoms, however minor, are interpreted as signs of cancer and panic attacks may occur. As with any other phobic disorder, cancer phobia cannot be treated by appeals to the reason.

The cause of phobias remains obscure but it seems likely that they are simple, forgotten conditioned reflexes which are kept active (*reinforced*) by the repeated drive to avoid the unpleasant experience. This view is supported by the success of behaviour therapy in removing phobias. The physiological responses to phobias – fast pulse, sweating, high blood pressure, and so on, can be controlled by the use of beta-blocking drugs.

## Pica

This is a persistent tendency to eat non-nutritional substances such as earth, ice, match-heads, coal, chalk or wood. Pica is common in children under 18 months of age and, in these, is not considered abnormal. Pica in pregnancy has been known throughout the ages and the bizarre catalogue of substances eaten include mothballs, soap, insects, clay, baking soda and excrement. Pica is a feature of nutritional deficiency and iron-deficiency anaemia and sometimes succeeds in providing a needed supply of minerals. It will often stop if anaemia is effectively treated.

In most cases, pica does little harm, but there have been many medical reports of obstruction or perforation of the bowel, lead poisoning, parasite infestation and other misfortunes from this cause. No satisfactory explanation of many types of pica has been produced.

## Plastic surgery
See COSMETIC SURGERY.

## PMT

See PERIOD PROBLEMS.

## Pregnancy

Pregnancy begins when a sperm enters an ovum and ends 266 to 270 days later when the baby is delivered. This is about 40 weeks from the first day of the last menstrual period. If fertilization has occurred too near the point where the FALLOPIAN TUBE enters the UTERUS there may be insufficient time for the ovum to develop to the stage at which it can implant in the lining of the UTERUS (*endometrium*). In this case, the pregnancy ends at that point.

About a week after entry of the sperm, the fertilized ovum becomes implanted in the endometrium, usually in the upper part, which has been prepared by the hormone stimulation from the *corpus luteum* of the ovary. Ultrasound scans can detect that the fetus is alive at six weeks but may not detect a fetal heartbeat at this stage in all cases.

### Pregnancy tests

These are tests, on urine or blood, to determine whether a living embryo or fetus is present within your body. Test kits are available from any chemist so that the test can be done at home. The tests depend on demonstrating the presence of human chorionic gonadotrophin, an ovary-stimulating hormone produced by the placenta. Immunological tests to detect the hormone by its combination with pre-prepared specific antibodies to it, can confirm pregnancy one or two weeks after the first missed menstrual period, or even earlier. The accuracy is nearly 100% if the test is positive, but about 80% if negative.

### Signs of pregnancy

Absence of menstruation is the most obvious sign. Most women have some nausea and vomiting in early pregnancy, known as morning sickness but not necessarily occurring in the mornings. This usually settles by about 12 weeks. Because the UTERUS lies close to the bladder, increasing size often causes increased frequency of the wish to empty the bladder. The breasts become engorged and enlarged and are often sore. There may be unusual tiredness. Progressive enlargement of the UTERUS and the detection of the fetal heartbeat with a Doppler instrument from about 12 weeks and with a stethoscope, at about the 24th week, are positive signs. Ultrasound scanning, which shows the fetal outline, can detect pregnancy, and determine viability, at about six weeks. X-rays which show the fetal skeleton are considered a positive sign of pregnancy. X-rays are, of course, normally avoided in pregnancy.

The areola of the BREAST is the pink or brown area surrounding the nipple. It is originally rose pink, but turns brown in the second month of the first pregnancy and never again regains its pristine hue. It contains tiny bumps (*tubercles*) under which are the areolar glands which lubricate the skin to protect it during suckling.

'Quickening' is the term given to the stage of pregnancy at which the mother-to-be first becomes aware of the movements of the fetus in her UTERUS. This commonly occurs at about the 18th week in a first pregnancy and about two weeks earlier in later pregnancies. By this time the uterus has enlarged enough to be in contact with the inside of the wall of the abdomen so that impulses are transmitted to the touch receptors near the surface. The sensations are, at first, feeble and barely perceptible and are often confused with 'wind', but as the fetus matures and its jerky movements increase in strength, the source of the sensation ceases to be in doubt.

Quickening is not a reliable sign of pregnancy. A woman anxious to conceive may easily become convinced that she is feeling fetal movements, when, in fact, she is not pregnant.

## The stages of pregnancy

For convenience, pregnancy is divided into three three-month periods called *trimesters*. By the end of the first trimester all the fetal body organs have begun to be formed and the fingers, toes, external genitalia, facial features and ears are visible. Damage from toxic agents, viruses and drugs are most serious during this period as they have the greatest effect.

During the second trimester, the fetal heart sounds become audible and the fetus can be felt through the abdominal wall. The growth of the uterus, with pressure on the abdominal organs, brings problems such as heartburn to the mother. Irregular contractions of the uterus, readily felt by the mother, occur. The fetal organs begin to function; blood vessels become visible through the transparent skin; and bones become more solid and conspicuous. Scalp hair begins to grow.

Uterus contractions become more frequent in the third trimester and all the symptoms due to a growing increase in pressure within the abdomen worsen. Upward pressure on the diaphragm limits full expansion of the lungs and causes breathlessness. During this trimester, the growth rate of the fetus is maximal and all normal external features of a baby, such as fingernails and toenails, testicles and ear lobes, become visible. *Lightening* is the sense of relief from abdominal fullness and discomfort commonly occurring in the last month of pregnancy when the baby's head settles down into the pelvic cavity. Lightening allows freer action of the diaphragm so that breathing is easier, but the pressure on the bladder and rectum may be worse. It may not occur with second or subsequent pregnancies as the head may not engage until the onset of labour.

**Multiple pregnancy**
This can result from fertilization of more than one ovum (non-identical twins) or from fertilization and egg division, followed by separation of the divided parts (identical twins). Triplets usually occur from a combination of these possibilities. Complications of pregnancy, especially prematurity, are commoner in multiple than in single pregnancies. The other complications, noted below are also commoner.

**Pregnancy complications**
Any process as complicated and busy as pregnancy might be expected to have something go wrong. The remarkable thing is that pregnancies are, on the whole, free from trouble.

**Vomiting in pregnancy**
Vomiting in early pregnancy is so common as to be considered almost normal. At least 50% of pregnant women are affected enough to complain. It usually begins by the sixth week and goes on until about the 12th week, but may continue throughout the pregnancy. It very rarely causes any danger to health. Although commonly known as 'morning sickness',

vomiting can occur at any time of the day and may be precipitated by travel, emotional stress or large meals of fatty food. Pregnancy sickness is probably caused by the action of unusual hormone levels on the vomiting centres in the brain, settling when these become habituated. Surprisingly, mere admission to hospital, without treatment, is often sufficient to stop excessive vomiting in pregnancy.

In about one case in 500, pregnancy vomiting becomes dangerously severe. This is called *hyperemesis gravidarum*. Excessive vomiting, and the associated low calorie intake, leads to a rise in the level of acetone-like substances in the blood (*ketosis*) and this prompts further vomiting by stimulating the vomiting centre in the brain. The condition may progress to a state of dehydration, alteration in the acidity of the blood, and liver damage. Urgent treatment, to restore fluid levels and control vomiting, is essential, as the condition is potentially fatal. Hyperemesis also threatens the fetus.

### Ectopic pregnancy

If the fertilized egg implants anywhere other than in the lining of the UTERUS (*endometrium*), an ectopic pregnancy results. This occurs in about one pregnancy in 200 and is especially likely if the FALLOPIAN TUBES have been affected by inflammation. By far the commonest site for an ectopic pregnancy is in a fallopian tube. Rarely, ectopics can occur in an OVARY or even within the abdominal cavity. Early diagnosis and surgical treatment are essential. Untreated ectopic pregnancies often end fatally from uncontrollable haemorrhage and surgical shock.

Ectopic pregnancy usually starts with cramping pain, and slight vaginal bleeding occurs soon after the first missed period. These are much more likely to be indications of threat-ened abortion (MISCARRIAGE) than ectopic pregnancy, but if they are followed by lower abdominal pain, localized to one side, and a deterioration in the general condition, you could be in danger. Urgent hospital management is needed. Gynaecological examination, blood and urine tests and ultra-sound scanning and laparoscopy, can establish the diagnosis, and surgical removal of the mass can be done immediately. This may involve removal of a length of fallopian tube, but every effort is made to preserve continuity and function, so that subsequent pregnancy is possible.

### Rubella

A maternal infection with German measles (*rubella*), in the first trimester of pregnancy can spread to the fetus. The rubella virus in the fetal tissues will cause a range of serious abnor-malities including congenital heart disease, congenital cataracts, congenital deafness, mental retardation and defects in the skeleton in up to 90% of babies. Lesser degrees of dam-age can occur from rubella later in pregnancy, but the more fully developed the organs the less the likelihood of damage.

For these reasons it is important that babies should have the combined measles, mumps, rubella vaccination. Failing this pre-pubertal girls and women who have never had rubel-la should be vaccinated. In Britain the Department of Health recommends that all girls should be vaccinated between their 10th and 14th birthdays. Tragedies have occurred because girls believed wrongly that they had had rubella. All women should be screened for rubella antibodies in every pregnancy. If you plan to get pregnant, insist on having a rubella antibody check first. Vaccination should never be done during pregnancy, however, as it is thought possible that the vaccine can affect the fetus. If there is a risk of pregnancy, effective contraception should be used for three months after vaccination.

### Pre-eclampsia

Eclampsia is a dangerous condition affecting pregnant women, in which major epileptic seizures (fits) and kidney damage occur and which carries a maternal mortality of about 3% and a baby death rate of about 15%. Eclampsia must be avoided at all costs. An important reason for antenatal examination is that it provides the opportunity for the detection of certain signs known to herald eclampsia. The combination of these signs is called pre-eclampsia.

The most important warning sign is a rise in the blood pressure. The other signs are the presence of protein in the urine – this is always abnormal – and the occurrence of excessive fluid retention in the tissues (*oedema*). If these signs are detected, or even if raised blood pressure, alone, occurs, a particularly close watch is maintained, often in hospital, and, if necessary, labour induced. The aim is to produce a live baby, as mature as possible, while preventing injury to the mother. If at all possible, the pregnancy is maintained until the 36th week. Rest in bed is an important measure. Drugs to reduce blood pressure are avoided if possible, as they may interfere with the blood supply to the fetus through the placenta. Imminent eclampsia is a signal for energetic measures to sedate the mother, get the blood pressure down and deliver the baby as soon as possible, often by CAESAREAN SECTION.

## PREGNANCY COMPLICATIONS

### Uterine fluid excess

This condition, known as hydramnios, is an abnormal increase in the volume of amniotic fluid in the pregnant UTERUS. The normal volume is about 800 ml and in hydramnios this may rise to well over two litres. In most cases the excess occurs gradually and is not noted until about the 30th week. Hydramnios occurs in about one pregnancy in 250. Often the cause is unknown, but the condition may occur if, for any reason, the fetus is unable to swallow amniotic fluid. This can occur if the fetal gullet (*oesophagus*) is abnormally narrowed. It is also common in the congenital abnormality in which the brain is absent (*anencephaly*).

Hydramnios may lead to premature rupture of the membranes and the umbilical cord may partly come out. Because of the increased freedom of movement of the fetus, abnormal positions of birth (*malpresentations*) are more common. There is also an increased risk of premature separation of the afterbirth (*placenta*).

Ultrasound examination will show if there are serious abnormalities in the fetus and the pregnancy may then be terminated. If there is great discomfort near term, labour may be induced. Some obstetricians believe that the removal of some of the fluid, by way of a needle passed through the abdominal wall, makes delivery safer.

### Cervical incompetence

Some women have repeated, painless, spontaneous MISCARRIAGES around the fourth or fifth month of pregnancy, and this may be due to the inability of the inner opening of the neck (*cervix*) of the UTERUS to remain properly closed. This is called cervical incompetence and it is usually, but not always, due to previous damage during delivery or to previous surgery. Such women, even when not pregnant, have an unusually wide cervix.

The treatment of this distressing condition is to insert a 'purse-string' circular stitch (*suture*) of non-absorbable material before the 16th week of pregnancy, but after the 12th week, when most spontaneous miscarriages have already occurred. This suture holds everything tight until the baby is almost due, when it is easily removed so that delivery can proceed.

### Antepartum haemorrhage

This is any bleeding from the UTERUS after about the 24th week of pregnancy. It may be due to an abnormality in the position, or the adequacy of attachment, of the placenta and occurs in about 3% of pregnancies. There may be a risk to the fetus from inadequate blood supply. If severe bleeding occurs, there may also be a risk to the mother. Fetal monitoring and a careful watch on the condition of both mother and baby is necessary. An emergency CAESAREAN SECTION may be required to save the baby.

### Malpresentation

Before birth, the baby normally lies head down with the chin tucked in and the back of the head to the front. Malpresentation exists if the baby lies in any other position, such as a bottom-first (*breech*) presentation, a transverse lie or a presentation with the neck extended instead of flexed and the back of the head to the rear.

Malpresentations may cause difficulty in, or even hold-up of, labour, and it may be necessary to try to turn the baby in the UTERUS (*version*) or to deliver by CAESARIAN SECTION. Internal version calls for great skill and is not without danger to the baby.

## Baby blues

A colourful Americanism for the misery and tearfulness which affect about half of all pregnant women, especially those having their first baby. The term is sometimes inaccurately applied to the distressing condition of pathological sadness (*puerperal depression*) which sometimes affects mothers soon after the birth. Baby blues usually starts suddenly and without warning on the second or third day after delivery and is usually over in about two months. In most cases, the depression is not severe, but in about one case in 1000 the condition becomes serious enough to require admission to hospital. Proper supervision and treatment of these serious cases is essential, for there is often a real risk of suicide or murder of the baby. Real depression should never be assumed just to be 'baby blues'.

## Prolapse

The displacement, often downwards, of the whole or part of an organ, from its normal position. Prolapse occurs because of weakness or laxity of some supporting structures, such as muscles or tendons. The commonest examples of prolapse are of the rectum and UTERUS, but the bladder may prolapse into the VAGINA; a haemorrhoid may prolapse through the anus; or the umbilical cord may prolapse from the uterus during or before birth.

## Protruding eyes

See EXOPHTHALMOS.

# R

## Rape

The British definition of rape is 'Sexual intercourse with a woman who does not, at the time, consent to it, by a man who knows she does not, or who is reckless as to whether or not she does'. The offence requires that there should have been some penetration of the VAGINA with the penis, however slight, but does not require that there should have been ejaculation of semen. Rape need not be forcible and can be effected by a trick, such as by impersonating a husband. Marriage is no defence to rape.

In some American States, the definition has been broadened to include other forms of sexual contact and to include acts against wives and acts by women against males. In the USA, statutory rape is sexual intercourse with a person below a specified age, which may vary in different states from 12 to 18. Intercourse with a mentally deficient or unconscious person may also be statutory rape. In Britain, such offences as these are described as 'sexual offences'.

Rape is not, as is often supposed, solely the result of ungovernable sexual urge. It is often motivated by anger and aggression against a person, a sex or a class, and often the rape victim becomes the symbol or scapegoat. Some rapists act to gratify sadistic impulses and often inflict cruel physical pain in association with the act.

Rape is still under-reported, but there is now a strong movement towards better understanding of the plight of the rape victim and sympathy for her. As a result, women are encouraged to report more assaults and to bring about prosecutions. Knowledge is growing, too, of the psychological effects of rape and of how these effects are best dealt with. SEXUALLY TRANSMITTED DISEASES and pregnancies resulting from rape are easily managed nowadays, but the associated mental distress, even with the highest standard of care, may be severe and prolonged.

Regrettably, unthinking prejudice against raped women still persists among many men, often with the explicit or implicit suggestion that women do not suffer rape unless they 'ask for it'. Only proper education of the young can undermine these damaging and uncivilized values.

## Rhesus factor disease

After the A,B, AB and O blood groups, the rhesus factor is the most important. The gene that makes a person rhesus positive is called D. This is present in 85% of the population. The gene is dominant, so a person is rhesus positive even if only one of the gene pair is D. All the offspring of a rhesus positive father with two D genes (*homozygous*) will be rhesus positive. If the father has only one D gene (*heterozygous*) and the mother is rhesus negative, each pregnancy will have a 50% chance of producing a rhesus positive baby.

When a rhesus positive father produces a rhesus positive baby in a rhesus negative mother, the baby's red blood cells will act as antigens capable of causing the mother to produce antibodies against them. These antigens do not normally reach the mother's blood until labour so they are unlikely to cause serious harm in the first pregnancy. But in subsequent pregnancies, the levels of these antibodies in the mother's blood rise rapidly and soon reach a point at which they are able to destroy the red cells of the fetus.

The severity of the effects on the baby vary considerably. In the most severe cases, the fetus dies in the UTERUS, usually after the 28th week. If born alive, the child may be deeply jaundiced with an enlarged liver and spleen and a low haemoglobin level in the red blood cells (*anaemia*). Excess free haemoglobin in the blood leads to excess bile pigment (*bilirubin*) production and this has a much more serious effect than merely to stain the skin and cause jaundice. Bilirubin is very toxic to the brain, which becomes bile-stained (*kernicterus*) and leads to paralysis, spasticity, mental retardation and defects of sight and hearing.

A badly affected baby can have an exchange transfusion, via the umbilical cord, as soon as it is born, or even while still in the uterus. This corrects the anaemia and gets rid of the bilirubin. Exposure to intense blue light soon after birth assists in converting the bilirubin in the skin to a form which is harmless to the brain.

Rhesus negative women can be prevented from developing antibodies by being given an injection of anti D gamma globulin within 60 hours of the birth of a rhesus positive baby. In order to protect future babies, this is done in all such cases. Gamma globulin is also given when there has been a MISCARRIAGE or if there is any other reason to believe that rhesus positive fetal blood may have gained access to the woman's circulation, as in obstetrical procedures like turning the baby (*external version*). The injection is given if an AMNIOCENTESIS shows bloodstained amniotic fluid, and is routine after an amniocentesis in a rhesus negative woman.

## Rubella

See PREGNANCY.

# S

## Sanitary protection

Materials or articles used to avoid bloodstaining of clothing during the menstrual period. In the past, women used rags which were washed and re-used. Today, a variety of disposable sanitary pads or intravaginal tampons are available, designed for light, moderate or heavy blood loss. Most women use between 15 and 20 tampons or pads a month.

Modern sanitary pads are made from layers of absorbent materials, such as paper and artificial cotton wool, enclosed in a surrounding layer of fabric. Discreet, self-adhesive pads which are designed to fit securely into close-fitting underpants have largely replaced oldfashioned belts and looped pads. The disadvantages of sanitary pads are that they sometimes chafe the inner thighs and may show under tight fitting clothes. Pads must be changed every four to six hours during the first few days of bleeding or they may become offensive.

A tampon is a cylinder of absorbent fibrous material inserted temporarily into the VAGINA to absorb menstrual blood and allow relatively unrestricted activity during the menstrual period. Tampons may also be used after surgical procedures on the neck of the UTERUS (*cervix*). Tampons have the advantage of being inconspicuous and can be worn for swimming. They can be used by women who have not had sexual intercourse, but insertion may be difficult. Tampons may be better for women prone to thrush, which thrives in the moist environment produced by a pad. Occasionally, a tampon is accidentally left in the VAGINA at the end of a period.

This may be a cause of VAGINAL DISCHARGE. Heavy staphylo-coccal infection of tampons is one of the causes of the TOXIC SHOCK SYNDROME.

## Scar removal

Many people have the idea that plastic surgeons have some magic way of closing skin without leaving scars. This, regret-tably, is a contradiction in terms. Skin heals by scar tissue and cannot heal otherwise. What the plastic surgeon tries to do is to make scars as thin and white as possible, to place them in the most inconspicuous positions and to ensure that they do not pull on tissue in an unnatural way.

Disfiguring scars, resulting from accidental injury or even, regrettably, from previous surgery, are unacceptable because they are broad, livid, deeply sunken, puckered and drag other areas of skin in the wrong direction. Time, alone, is one of the best treatments for such scars and a surprising improvement nearly always occurs, over the course of several months, fol-lowing severe incised wounds of the skin. But ugly scars do persist and much can be done, by cosmetic surgery, to improve the appearance.

The surgeon will start by studying the scar, noting its qual-ity, depth and the direction in which it runs. He or she will note whether this direction crosses any of the natural lines of the skin and whether there is any distortion of proper skin dis-position or puckering. A detailed plan of action is important and this will take into account the necessity to cut out all dense, broad and deep scar tissue and then bring together the skin edges in such a way that the new scar entirely relieves tension and does not, itself, cause disfigurement.

An ugly, straight and deep scar is likely to end up as a faint zigzag, some of the lines of which will lie in natural skin creases and will be almost invisible. A technique called Z-*plasty* is commonly used to achieve this, and a skilled and imaginative surgeon can do wonders in altering the lines of tension in the skin by this means. The Z-plasty idea has been extended and there is now a remarkable range of tricks which can be applied in the revision of scars. Skin grafting is seldom necessary for wound scars and this is fortunate, for it is difficult to get an accurate match with skin taken from any other site. Extensive scars, such as those caused by burns, may, of course, require grafting.

## Sexual problems

Sexual activity encompasses physical, psychological, social and aesthetic elements. Anything as complex as this is liable to a range of disorders. These disorders may be apparent only to one member of a partnership or to both, and may be attributed by either to the other or to the unsatisfactory nature of the relationship. The latter is one of the most common causes of trouble. It is unreasonable to expect a good sexual rapport between people who dislike one another or who are concerned primarily with their own personal satisfaction rather than with that of the other. Fear of pregnancy, sexual ignorance, and guilt induced by misinformation and religious instruction are other major causes of sexual problems.

The proportion of sexual problems attributable to organic or structural disorder is small: the great majority are of psychological or inter-relational origin. They include:

- impotence
- ejaculatory disorders, especially premature ejaculation
- lack of orgasm in females
- inability to relax the muscles of the genitalia (VAGINISMUS)
- various forms of sexual deviation

Organic disease such as neurologically- or diabetically-induced impotence, penile distortion (*Peyronie's disease*) in males, or VAGINAL DRYNESS or shrinkage of the VAGINA in the elderly woman, can cause serious sexual difficulties.

### Painful sexual intercourse

The medical term for this is dyspareunia, a word that derives from the Greek *dyspareunos* meaning 'ill-mated'. This is a little hard on the woman who is usually suffering from a gynaeco-logical disorder such as an imperforate or thick, persistent hymen, vulvitis, vaginitis, bartholinitis, urethritis, episiotomy scars, vaginal dryness, senile or post-radiational atrophy of the VAGINA, or, rarely, a congenital central vaginal partition (*septate*, or double, vagina).

Dyspareunia is often caused by vaginal spasm (*vaginismus*) which may be of such degree that even a finger can barely be admitted. This condition is of psychological origin and is usu-ally caused by fear of sex or by disinclination for sexual inter-course with a particular partner. Vaginismus is a major reflex spasm, which may involve not only all the muscles of the pelvis, but also the muscles which press the thighs together. Treatment is often difficult and may, in some cases, be inap-propriate. Psychotherapy, skilled counselling and patient explanation, relaxation training, genital self-familiarization, and the use, by the affected woman, of progressively larger smooth, rounded dilators, may be needed. What is *not* needed is male assertiveness and force. This causes pain, and exacerbates the basic causal factors.

**Non-consummation**
This means failure to achieve penetration of the vagina with the penis. This is commoner than is generally supposed and is believed to be the fate of about one marriage in 100.

Non-consummation occasionally results from ignorance on the part of both partners, remarkable in these outspoken days, as to what should go where. More commonly, it results from physical or psychological problems. The man may suffer impotence, of whatever sort, failure to maintain the erection, premature ejaculation or penile abnormality. The woman may have an anatomical abnormality of the vagina or a thick, rigid hymen, or, most commonly, the condition of vaginismus (see above).

## Sexually transmitted diseases
These used to be called venereal diseases, but since the word *venereal* means 'relating to love', the present term is probably more appropriate. The range of sexually transmitted diseases is wider than most people realize, and there has been a change in their pattern of occurrence over the last three or four decades. The figures for syphilis are continuing to drop and, fortunately, this unpleasant disease has now become much less common than it used to be. Only about 2,000 cases are reported each year, in Britain, and it is now really only a problem in the homosexual community. Syphilis acquired before birth (*congenital syphilis*) is now very rare. On the other hand,

genital herpes is booming. Its prevalence has increased faster than that of any other sexually transmitted disease. Chlamydial infections – most cases of *non-specific urethritis* are chlamydial – are also flourishing. They are well up at the top of the list.

Gonorrhoea, popularly known as 'the clap', once the scourge of the promiscuous, seems to be falling back a little. The gonococcus, however, has, for years, been developing resistance to penicillin, a drug which was once was a 100% sure cure. Much larger doses of penicillin are now needed than formerly, and doctors are always worried about the emergence of strains of the organism which are totally resistant to ordinary penicillin. These strains were first noted in 1976 and the number of cases caused by the totally resistant strains has doubled each year since then.

Thrush (*candidiasis*), although not necessarily a sexually transmitted disease, is very commonly spread by sexual intercourse, and the figures are only a little lower than those for gonorrhoea. Genital warts and trichomoniasis are flourishing. Again, the trichomonas is not necessarily sexually spread. That leaves a miscellaneous group of infestations including crab lice, scabies and infections such as Gardnerella vaginalis infection, molluscum contagiosum, lymphogranuloma venereum, chancroid and yaws. Some of these occur only in the tropics.

Sexually transferred hepatitis is steadily becoming more common. Worst of all is the acquired immune deficiency syndrome (AIDS) whose incidence has been doubling yearly since it appeared in 1981. AIDS has become increasingly a woman's problem as the number of infected people increases. It started among certain homosexual men simply because they were, at the time, the only group promiscuous enough to build up a critical level of the HIV in a society. There are now heterosexual communities in which such levels are being reached. In these, promiscuous heterosexual women are as much at risk as promiscuous homosexual or heterosexual men. See AIDS.

This increase in sexually transmitted diseases suggest that they are difficult to avoid. This is true for people engaging in regular promiscuous sexual activity who will certainly, sooner or later, and probably sooner rather than later, acquire a sexually transmitted disease. The question is whether the disease is just a minor annoyance, easily cured, or whether it is one which seriously, and perhaps permanently, affects health.

Sexually transmitted disease is never just simply a matter of physical health, like picking up a bad cold or appendicitis. Sexually acquired disease, by definition, involves some other person, and questions of blame, and often recrimination, will usually arise. Third parties – perhaps an innocent spouse – may be involved. Normal people will inevitably feel guilt or deep resentment and even if the latter is not openly expressed, its effect is bound to be damaging to the relationship.

Many people react to the discovery that they have a sexually transmitted disease by losing interest in sexual intercourse, especially with the person from whom the disease was acquired. Some people become very angry when they find that they have acquired a sexually transmitted disease and some become violent. These are major problems having an important bearing on health in the wider sense. Relationships are of basic importance to health and happiness and anything that damages them is dangerous and damaging to us all.

## Herpes

Genital herpes is caused by the herpes simplex virus and most cases are caused by type 2 virus, which is a slightly different strain from the type 1 virus that causes cold sores. Some people, however, for obvious reasons, get sexually transmitted herpes from the type 1 virus and cold sores from type 2.

The first sign of genital herpes appears within one week of exposure. This is a red, painful rash which appears on the vulva or on the surrounding skin. The rash may be confined to the genital area or may be more widespread, involving the thighs or buttocks. The more widespread the rash, the more severe the pain. Soon the rash develops blisters and these progress to ulcers which may join up to form quite large areas of ulceration with shallow cratering. At this stage, the sores are very sensitive, and passing urine may be extremely uncomfortable. There are often enlarged and tender glands in the groin, showing that the infection has spread deeply into the body. Some people have slight fever and general illness. Finally, about three weeks after the beginning of the attack, the ulcers crust over and begin to heal. The pain usually goes away about two weeks after the rash first appears.

About four months after infection, the first recurrence usually appears. This is often preceded, for about two days, by a local tingling sensation with excessive sensitivity of the skin in the areas about to be affected. Recurrences are hardly ever as severe as the first attack and do not last as long. The new blisters usually heal in just under two weeks from the time of appearance. At all times when any blisters or rash are present, the affected person is highly infectious to others. Many people

find that recurrences of herpes are brought on by menstruation, stress, sexual intercourse or other factors.

At present it seems that herpes is probably not curable.
Once the virus is established in the body, indefinite recurrences are likely. The drug acyclovir is very helpful, but there
is little evidence that it can completely cure the infection. It is
certainly by far the most effective treatment, to date, in reducing the severity of the disease and shortening the duration of
attacks. It is apparently quite safe and can be taken in large
doses either by mouth or, in very severe cases, by injection.
Research work is proceeding apace both in the modification of
acyclovir, so as to make it more effective, and in the hunt for
new, similar drugs.

## Chlamydial infection and gonorrhoea

The commonest early signs of these sexually transmitted diseases are vaginal and urethral discharges and severe irritation.
These symptoms occur two to five days after intercourse in
the case of gonorrhoea, and seven to 21 days in the case of
chlamydia. Vaginal discharge is, of course, very common and
most cases are not sexually transmitted. But a change in the
character of the discharge, especially one occurring a few days
after a new sexual contact, is likely to mean trouble.

Gonorrhoea and chlamydial disease start as an infection of
the neck of the UTERUS (*cervix*) and, unfortunately, in about half
the cases, the woman concerned may be unaware that anything untoward has happened. In about 10% of cases, the
infection spreads up into the uterus and along the FALLOPIAN
TUBES, where it causes inflammation known as salpingitis. This
can lead to blockage, with sterility, or partial blockage with

the risk of a pregnancy occurring in the tube (*ectopic pregnancy*). Repeated attacks of gonorrhoea or chlamydial infection are likely to cause permanent sterility. After three or more attacks, about three-quarters of women have totally blocked tubes.

The organisms causing these conditions often spread further to cause persistent inflammation of the inside of the pelvis and there may be constant, dragging abdominal pain, tenderness and fever. In addition, there is likely to be discomfort, or even pain, on sexual intercourse. Occasionally abscesses occur in the LABIA.

In the early stages, both gonorrhoea and chlamydial infections are easily treated with antibiotics, the former with one of the penicillins and the latter with a tetracycline. Given in proper dosage and under skilled supervision these treatments are very effective and a cure is usual. But once the secondary complications have developed, treatment is much more difficult and much less sure. Surgical operations may sometimes be necessary in the treatment of chronic pelvic inflammation and even this may be unsuccessful.

## Syphilis

This disease is quite rare in women. Most new cases occur in homosexual males. The condition, which is caused by the spirochaete *Treponema pallidum*, appears about three weeks after exposure, but the period from contact to onset (*incubation period*) may be as long as three months. The first sign is the chancre. This is a single, small, red area, slightly raised and entirely painless, occurring on any part of the vulva or even on the cervix of the UTERUS. The chancre is sometimes so inconspicuous that it can be missed entirely, with dire consequences. After a few days the raised area ulcerates, still painlessly, to leave a clean, round wet crater with a hardened edge and base and teeming with spirochaetes. Within three to ten weeks the chancre has healed. The glands in the groin often enlarge and feel rubbery, but there is no pain or tenderness.

The secondary stage starts four to eight weeks after the appearance of the chancre, and, if the chancre has been missed, provides another chance of appreciating that something serious has happened. The commonest feature of secondary syphilis is a skin rash of circular spots, up to 1 cm in diameter and either rosy pink or coppery red, scattered over the chest, back, abdomen and arms. These spots are painless and not even itchy so they have to be looked for. In areas where two layers of skin are in contact these spots may expand and become large and fleshy (*condylomata lata*), and on the lips or in the mouth or on the genitalia shallow, painless ulcers, resembling snail tracks, may form. Even if nothing is done, these signs will eventually disappear and the uninformed or unwary may think that that is the end of the matter.

In six out of ten people with untreated syphilis nothing much more happens. But in the other 40% several very unpleasant things may occur. The late effects of syphilis may be delayed for many years, but if they occur they do so with a vengeance. They include:

- ballooning and fatal bursting of the major artery of the body (*aneurysm of the aorta*)
- neurological damage which may cause loss of sensation in

the feet and joints, blindness, incontinence, impotence, inability to maintain balance or several other grave misfortunes

- an organic psychiatric syndrome featuring personality changes, delusions of grandeur, severe defect of judgement and paralysis (*general paralysis of the insane*)

This is a fate on no account to be risked and people who suspect they may have contracted syphilis, however long before, should ask for a VDRL (*Venereal Disease Reference Laboratory*) test and, if necessary, antibiotic treatment – which, if things have not gone too far, is highly effective.

### Lymphogranuloma venereum

This sexually transmitted disease is also caused by *Chlamydia trachomatis,* and is widespread in the tropics. Cases occasionally occur in Britain.

One to five weeks after exposure a small ulcer appears on the genitalia, but soon heals. The lymph nodes in the groin soon become inflamed, enlarged and matted together and the overlying skin develops a dusky pink colour. Sometimes there is fever, headache, aches and pains, loss of weight, and, in a few cases, a rash and enlargement of the spleen.

If the infection is not treated, abscesses may form in the glands and these may ulcerate through to the surface leaving multiple discharging openings on the skin of the groins, which may take months to heal.

Treatment is with antibiotic drugs such as a tetracycline and this is effective.

## Skin cancer

Many skin cancers are related to long-term exposure to sunlight. This is especially so in the cases of basal cell carcinoma (*rodent ulcer*), squamous cell carcinoma, which may develop in an area of actinic keratosis, and malignant melanoma in white people. These three conditions occur in that order of frequency, but, fortunately, the commonest, the basal cell carcinoma, is the least malignant, and the rarest, the melanoma, the most serious. Bowen's disease, which is a very slow-growing cancer within the epidermis, may also be related to sunlight exposure.

About one cancer in a hundred is a malignant melanoma. Skin melanomas are very rare in childhood and are commonest in the middle-aged and the elderly. About half of them arise from pre-existing moles. Nearly everyone has pigmented moles but only one in a million becomes malignant. Hairy moles hardly ever turn into malignant melanomas.

Malignant change in a mole can be detected by various signs. These include:

- change in shape, especially increasing irregularity of outline
- change in size
- increased protuberance beyond the surface
- change in colour, especially sudden darkening and the development of coloured irregularities appearing as different shades of brown, grey, pink, red and bluish
- itching or pain
- softening
- crumbling

- the development of new 'satellite' moles around the original one

The most dangerous melanomas are those that become nodular. This is because these tend to penetrate deeply.

Melanomas are commonest on areas exposed to the sun, but may occur anywhere on the skin. Once your suspicion has been aroused, you should never delay reporting the condition for an expert opinion. Melanomas are removed with a wide area of normal-seeming tissue around them and skin grafting may be necessary to cover the defect.

## Skin disorders

The skin is at least as susceptible to disease as any other organ and the range of disorders is wide. The discipline dealing with skin disorders is called dermatology. The term *dermatitis* does not, as is commonly thought, refer to a particular condition. It simply means 'inflammation of the skin' and covers all skin disorders in which the skin is inflamed.

Many cases of dermatitis are caused by:

- infection by almost any kind of organism – viruses, bacteria, fungi and protozoa
- allergy to a wide range of contact materials
- physical or chemical injury
- damage by heat, intense ultraviolet light, or by other forms of radiation

The term *eczema* is roughly synonymous with *dermatitis*. Urticaria (*hives*) is the common skin reaction to allergy, whether from contact or ingestion.

Bacterial infection by staphylococci causes pustules, boils and carbuncles, and infection by streptococci causes spreading skin inflammation (*cellulitis*). Both staphylococci and streptococci can cause impetigo. Virus infections of the skin include cold sores and venereal herpes from herpes simplex viruses and most forms of warts. In shingles – herpes zoster – the virus is usually acquired early in life, when it causes chickenpox. Fungus infection, or epidermophytosis, causes the various forms of tinea – athlete's foot (*tinea pedis*), crutch infection (*tinea cruris*), body infection (*tinea corporis*) and ringworm of the scalp (*kerion*). Fungus also commonly infects the nails.

Infestation with various mite and insect parasites, such as the scabies mite, *Sarcoptes scabei*, fleas, bed bugs and lice, cause damage to the skin and this is often compounded by damage and secondary infection from scratching.

Birth-marks, or naevi, may take several different forms, including the port-wine stain caused by enlargement of capillaries (very small blood vessels) and pigmented moles. See also SKIN CANCER.

Common acne with the formation of blackheads (*comedones*) is related to the local action, on the sebaceous glands of the skin, of androgens (male sex hormones). A combined antiandrogen/oestrogen pill is often valuable in the management. Although it is not an infection, acne can be treated effectively a tetracycline antibiotic. Regular washing with soap and water and the use of a chlorhexidine scrub, such as Hibiscrub, are also helpful. The most effective treatment of all is the drug isotretinoin, but this can cause severe fetal abnormalities and young women who are proposing to use it must have a negative pregnancy test and must use an oral contraceptive for a month before the course, during it, and for three months afterwards.

A wen (*sebaceous cyst*) is an accumulation of sebaceous material within the skin, following the blockage of a pore.

A scar is an area of fibrous tissue which has replaced normal skin during the healing of a deep injury. Such fibrous tissue contracts on maturation, causing depression of the surface.

Psoriasis is a very common and persistent skin disease with a complex cause. It features well-demarcated, oval, reddish patches with scaly surfaces and may vary markedly in severity at different times.

XANTHELASMA features yellowish plaques in the skin due to deposition of cholesterol. These commonly occur in the eyelids and do not necessarily imply raised blood cholesterol levels.

Excessive BLUSHING may herald the condition of rosacea, in which the small blood vessels of the face have an abnormal tendency to dilate.

Purpura is a condition of leaky blood vessels so that blood is released into the tissues. In the skin this may cause tiny pinpoints or dots (*petechiae*) or larger bruises.

Vitiligo is characterized by pure white patches in the skin, particularly noticeable in non-white or suntanned people. It is believed to be caused by an autoimmune destruction of the pigment cells.

Prickly heat is caused by high temperatures and humidity which lead to blockage of the ducts of sweat glands, so that small papules form.

A common cause of acceleration of skin degeneration is

undue exposure to ultraviolet light. Sunbathing is a major cause of collagen damage with loss of skin elasticity and excessive wrinkling. Keratosis is also commonly caused by solar radiation and may lead to skin cancer. Other forms of radiation, such as X-rays, may cause severe injury to the skin and may eventually lead to cancer.

## Spider naevi

These common, tiny skin blemishes consist of small, central, slightly raised, bright red areas from which fine red lines radiate, like spider legs. A few spider naevi are of no import, but numerous spider naevi are commonly found in serious persistent liver disease, such as *cirrhosis*. They are also common in women receiving HORMONE REPLACEMENT THERAPY.

## Sterilization

This is usually done by closing off the FALLOPIAN TUBES. The operation is comparatively minor and is done using laparoscopic methods through very small incisions in the abdominal wall. The tubes may be tied and cut, or simply clamped with plastic rings. Alternatively, they may be burned through with an electric cautery and thus sealed.

Nearly 100,000 female sterilizations are done each year in Britain, usually as a permanent method of contraception. The failure rate is very low, but those that do fail carry a greatly increased risk of ECTOPIC PREGNANCY. Sterilization can usually be reversed, if this is desired. Success, in the sense of subsequent conception, occurs in about 75% of cases.

HYSTERECTOMY also implies sterilization, but this cannot be reversed.

## Stillbirth

This is the term used for the birth of a dead baby. The distinction between stillbirth and MISCARRIAGE is arbitrary and in Britain is set at 24 weeks of pregnancy. A baby at this stage is regarded as being viable and the birth and death must be registered. Before burial may take place, the cause of death must be established, if possible, sometimes by autopsy, and a certificate of stillbirth provided.

In many cases, the cause of death of the fetus is not established. Diabetes or high blood pressure in the mother, rhesus incompatibility, eclampsia, severe fetal malformations, inadequacy of the placenta, or infections such as toxoplasmosis, rubella, syphilis or herpes simplex are all well-recognized causes.

## Striae

Striae are broad lines, called stretch marks, on the skin of the abdomen, thighs and breasts. They are red at first and slightly raised, but later become purplish and flattened. About three quarters of pregnant women develop striae and, unfortunately, because they involve damage to the elastic collagen in the skin, striae are permanent. They do, however, become very much less obvious with the passage of time, and eventually are often barely visible.

## Suction lipectomy

This is a cosmetic operation to get rid of surplus fat under the skin. Small incisions are made through the skin at strategic points and through these are passed a blunt-ended metal tube (*cannula*) connected to a powerful vacuum pump. Because human fat is a liquid oil at body temperatures, and because the walls of the fat cells are thin and easily broken, the cannula can be moved around under the skin to break down cell walls and vacuum out unwanted fat. There is a variable degree of bruising from damage to blood vessels, and if your skin is stretched and lax, you may end up looking a little deflated. Needless to say, unless the procedure is accompanied by a radical change in eating habits, the body will soon revert to the status quo.

## Swallowing difficulty
See DYSPHAGIA.

## Sweating
See HYPERHIDROSIS.

## Swollen arm
See LYMPHOEDEMA.

# T

## Tamoxifen

Tamoxifen is a remarkable drug with a very persistent effect that prevents oestrogens from acting normally in the body. It has been in use since 1971 to help to treat breast cancer in over three million women. The drug delays relapse and prolongs survival in 20–30% of affected women. Many thousands of these women have survived for more than 10 years.

There is much current interest in whether the drug is effective in preventing high-risk women from developing breast cancer. Trials of the drug in the USA, Italy, Australia and Britain, suggest that it may be a valuable preventive. In women who have had one primary breast cancer the drug appears to reduce the incidence of a second cancer by about 40%. The anti-oestrogen effects appear, on the whole, to be beneficial rather than otherwise. Older women taking the drug enjoy a 60% reduction in death from heart attacks and are significantly protected against postmenopausal osteoporosis. Pre-menopausal women have not been found to suffer such effects as an early menopause, loss of sexual interest or VAGINAL DRYNESS. Some side effects are inevitable and some women taking the drug experience hot flushes, nausea, fluid retention, irregularity of menstruation and vaginal discharge. None of these effects should weigh heavily in the light of the advantages. Tamoxifen stimulates egg release (*ovulation*) and is often used in the treatment of infertility.

In Spring 1992 the American National Cancer Institute

recruited 16,000 healthy women, deemed to be at high risk of breast cancer, into a tamoxifen trial. Half of these women are acting as controls and are taking an inactive placebo; half are taking the active drug. None of them know whether what they are taking is the drug or the dummy. The trial is expected to last for five years. Some doctors have criticized trials of this kind, pointing out that tamoxifen is not as harmless as many suggest. The fact that large multinational trials are being mounted by people who are well aware of these risks does, however, suggest that the majority consider the risks worth taking.

## Tampon

See SANITARY PROTECTION.

## Thrush

Infection of warm, moist areas of the body with the common fungus of the genus *Candida*. Most cases are caused by the species *Candida albicans* which causes thrush of the mouth or VAGINA and occasionally elsewhere on the skin. Candida thrives best in darkness when the temperatures are right and especially when there is a good supply of carbohydrate for its nutrition. Candidiasis of the female vulva is thus particularly common if there is diabetes, in which there is sugar in the urine. So a urine test is mandatory in all such cases.

Fungus infections tend to be kept in check by the presence of normal body bacteria (*commensal organisms*) and if these are too energetically attacked by antibiotics, fungi may get the upper hand and start to spread.

Vaginal thrush is easily recognized. There is persistent

itching or soreness and sometimes a burning pain on contact between urine and affected areas. Inspection shows characteristic white patches, rather like soft cheese, with raw-looking inflamed areas in between. There may be a white, cheesy vaginal discharge. Vulval candidiasis is easily transmitted to a sexual partner, and men, especially if uncircumcized, often develop white patches and inflammation on the glans of the penis. This is called balanitis and there is constant discomfort, varying from mild to severe.

Apart from involvement of these areas, candidiasis is uncommon in otherwise healthy people. It flourishes, however, in people whose immune systems are in any way defective. In AIDS, candidiasis spreads widely both outside and inside the body, extending from the mouth and the anal region well into both ends of the intestinal tract. Even more seriously, it often spreads into the respiratory passages and the lungs.

Candidiasis is treated with one of a range of antifungal drugs in the form of ointments, creams, meltable bullets for insertion in the vagina (*pessaries*) or drugs taken by mouth. Anti-thrush drugs include Canesten (clotrimazole), Daktarin (miconazole), Nystan (nystatin) and Diflucan (fluconazole). Thrush can be cured with a single dose of the latter drug. Treating only one of a pair of sexual partners, however, is a waste of time. This has to be a joint effort.

## Thyroid function tests

The function of the thyroid gland is to synthesize the thyroid hormone – the iodine-containing amino acid, thyroxine (T4), which has four iodine atoms in each molecule, and tri-iodothyronine (T3) with three iodines per molecule. So the most direct way to test thyroid function is to measure the rate at which iodine is accumulated by the gland. This is conveniently done by using a radioactive isotope of iodine which, although chemically identical to the normal element, can easily be assessed by measuring the level of radioactivity at the gland with a radiation counter held in front of the neck. This is called thyroid scanning and the measurement is usually taken half an hour after administering a dose of the isotope by mouth. The amounts of the two hormones, T4 and T3, in the blood, can be measured in the laboratory using samples of serum taken from the patient.

Because the thyroid gland has such a marked influence on the metabolic rate, its function may be assessed by measurements of the rate of oxygen consumption in the resting state. This is called the basal metabolic rate (BMR), and its estimation was once widely used as a test of thyroid function. Other tests have now replaced BMR measurements.

The pituitary gland not only controls thyroid gland activity, but is also influenced by the levels of thyroid hormones in the blood. Thus, a measurement of the amount of thyroid stimulating hormone (TSH) produced by the pituitary gland can be a valuable indirect test of thyroid function.

## Thyroid gland disorders

Women are far more often troubled by thyroid gland disorders than men. This goes for both overaction and underaction of the gland. The thyroid hormones, thyroxine and tri-iodothyronine, act on all the cells in the body which are consuming energy, to speed up the processes of fuel consumption.

Normally, the amount of thyroid hormone in the blood is carefully controlled so that these metabolic processes occur at a correct rate. In thyroid overaction (*thyrotoxicosis*, or *hyperthyroidism*) there is excessive production of thyroid hormones, so that all these cellular processes are accelerated. In most cases the gland is either generally enlarged or contains many nodules of overactive thyroid tissue. The causes of thyrotoxicosis have not been fully explained.

Thyrotoxicosis causes:

- a marked speeding up of many of the bodily processes
- loss of weight in spite of good appetite and large intake
- rapid heart rate
- irregular pulse
- palpitation
- tremor
- sweating
- dislike of hot weather
- frequent bowel actions
- anxiety and inability to relax

A common feature is a staring appearance of the eyes, caused by a marked retraction of the upper lids. Sometimes, the eyes may protrude markedly (EXOPHTHALMOS) as a result of swelling of the tissues behind them, but this may occur long after the acute illness has subsided. THYROID FUNCTION TESTS show abnormal levels of the thyroid hormones in the blood.

Thyrotoxicosis is treated with drugs, such as carbimazole, methimazole and thiouracil, which cut down the activity of the gland, and sometimes by surgical removal of part of the gland (*partial thyroidectomy*). Gland activity can also be reduced by the use of a radioactive isotope of iodine. While treatment is having effect, many of the symptoms can be relieved by the use of beta-blocker drugs.

Underaction of the thyroid gland in the adult, usually the result of autoimmune diseases such as HASHIMOTO'S THYROIDITIS, is known as hypothyroidism. This features:

- an overall slowing of the physical and mental processes
- sensitivity to cold
- obesity
- absence of sweating with scaly dry skin
- loss of hair
- puffiness of the face
- premature ageing
- coronary artery disease
- an eventual descent, unless treatment is given, into immobility and coma

Thyroid hormone, given early enough, will restore normality.

Enlargement of the thyroid gland, from any cause, is called GOITRE. Some small degree of goitre often occurs, as a normal event, around puberty or during pregnancy, but this usually settles without treatment.

Thyroid cancer is comparatively rare and presents as a single firm lump in the neck around the Adam's apple (*larynx*). If more than one lump is felt, the condition is unlikely to be cancer, but all lumps in this area must be properly investigated. Cancers grow gradually to form an increasing, irregular mass which is adherent to the adjacent structures and which spreads quickly to the lymph nodes in the neck. The nerves supplying the muscles of the vocal cords in the larynx may be involved, causing severe hoarseness or loss of the voice. Spread of the cancer to the gullet (*oesophagus*) may cause difficulty in swallowing.

Thyroid cancer is treated by surgical removal, by giving thyroid hormone, which restricts tumour growth, or by the use of radioactive iodine, which concentrates in the thyroid gland and in any secondary deposits of thyroid cancer elsewhere in the body.

## Toxic shock syndrome

This is an acute, dangerous, but fortunately rare, condition caused by the absorption into the bloodstream of toxins (*toxaemia*) from bacteria of the *Staphylococcus aureus* species. An epidemic of the toxic shock syndrome occurred among young menstruating women in the early 1980s and the condition was found to be associated with high-absorbency vaginal tampons and a rise in the staphylococci in the VAGINA.

The organism *S. aureus* produces three different kinds of toxins and these produce three different syndromes – food poisoning, the *scalded skin syndrome* in newborn babies and small children, and the toxic shock syndrome. Ninety per cent of cases of the toxic shock syndrome occur in menstruating women. The others occur in people with severe staphylococcal infections of the bone or the heart valves, or following operations.

There is a fever of 40°C or above, an acute drop in blood pressure, a rash which becomes scaly, vomiting, diarrhoea, muscle pain, inflammation of the vagina, liver damage and sometimes disorientation and confusion. The mortality is about 2%.

Because the trouble is caused by the toxins which have already been released from the organisms, killing the staphylococci with antibiotics has little effect on the course of the illness. It does, however, reduce the likelihood of recurrence and such treatment is always given. The use of high absorbency tampons must be avoided and all tampons should be changed frequently. It is especially important to remove the last tampon at the end of a period.

## Trichomoniasis

A genital infection with the single-celled organism *Trichomonas vaginalis*. The infection is usually transmitted by sexual intercourse and most commonly affects the VAGINA, but may also involve the urine tube (*urethra*) in either sex and the prostate gland in men.

Trichomoniasis causes severe irritation, burning and itching and a frothy, yellowish, offensive discharge. It is one of the common causes of vaginal discharge. If the urethra is affected, there is burning on urination and some urethral discharge. Vaginal trichomoniasis often causes discomfort or pain during sexual intercourse.

Men with a prostatic infection can act as carriers of the infection and if one of a pair of sexual partners has the infection, both must be treated or no advantage will be gained. The drug Flagyl (metronidazole) is the mainstay of treatment and is highly effective. See also SEXUALLY TRANSMITTED DISEASES.

## Twins

Two offspring from a single pregnancy. The incidence of twins is about one in 90 pregnancies. Twins may be identical, if they both arise from one fertilized egg (ovum), or non-identical, if two separate ova are separately fertilized by separate spermatozoa.

Twins developing from a single ovum are called monozygotic or monovular twins and have identical genetic material. They occur if the fertilized ovum separates completely, at an early stage of development, into two embryos, each of which then proceeds to develop normally. Very rarely, this division occurs too late so that separation is incomplete, resulting in Siamese twins. Monozygotic twins are both nourished by the same single placenta. They may differ in size at birth, but are always of the same sex and appearance.

Twin pregnancies call for more intensive antenatal care than usual as they involve a somewhat higher incidence of complications such as pre-eclampsia, anaemia, excess amniotic fluid and congenital malformations. Women with twins are often admitted to hospital earlier than those with single pregnancies. They need more rest than average. Twins should always be delivered in hospital, because complications of labour, such as breech or other malpresentation, may occur and because resuscitation of the small babies may be necessary. It is usual to perform an episiotomy (see CHILDBIRTH) to protect the head of the small babies.

Having twins imposes a considerable additional burden on the mother. Twins do not preclude BREASTFEEDING and many mothers find this more convenient than bottlefeeding. It is certainly better for the babies, and the smaller they are the more they benefit from it.

# U

## Ultrasound scanning

Unlike electromagnetic radiations such as X-rays and gamma rays which pass easily through a vacuum, sound is a vibration of the molecules of a gas, liquid or solid. Vibrations between about sixteen cycles per second (hertz) and twenty thousand cycles per second are perceptible as sound, but we are deaf to those of a higher frequency. Audible sound waves have long wavelengths – often several metres long – and can only be reflected by very large surfaces, such as the side of a mountain, causing echoes. The higher the frequency of the vibration, the shorter the wavelength and the smaller the area needed for reflection.

In ultrasound scanning, a beam of 'sound' – of a frequency of about three to ten million cycles per second – is projected into the body. Whenever it meets a surface between tissues of different density, echoes are created and these return to the source. The time taken to do so depends on the distance. The ultrasound waves are produced by feeding short pulses of alternating current, at the frequency desired, to a piezoelectric crystal in the scanner head. The electrical variations cause the crystal to vibrate at the same frequency. Piezoelectric materials have the property of working in both directions – they change shape when electricity is applied to them, but they also generate electricity if their shape is distorted. So the returning echoes cause the crystal to act as a microphone and this, in turn, generates a tiny electric current. The length of time between the emitted pulse and the returning echo is a measure of the distance to the interface. Any device which converts one mode of energy into another is called a *transducer* and this is the term used for the scanner head.

The ultrasound is focused into a narrow parallel beam which is scanned from side to side in one plane of the body. The returning echoes are correlated, in a computer, with the corresponding angle of the beam, and this enables a two-dimensional picture to be built up. Developments of great sophistication have produced ever higher resolution and improvement in the standards of the display. Even so, ultrasound scans are still only representations of interfaces and require to be interpreted by experts. The quality is much less good than that of computer assisted tomography (CT) scans or magnetic resonance imaging (MRI) and it is mainly their high safety that recommends them.

So far as is known, ultrasound, of the intensity and frequency used in scanning, is completely harmless. There are no recorded instances in the literature of any damage being caused. Millions of pregnant women have had scans with no indications of harm to the fetus or mother. Ultrasound of higher intensity can cause tissue warming and is sometimes used for treatment purposes by physiotherapists.

One of the principal uses of ultrasound scanning is in obstetrics. Today, the majority of pregnant women are screened by ultrasound, usually around the 16th to 18th week of pregnancy. Ultrasound can detect twins, can confirm that the fetus is of a size appropriate to the stage of pregnancy, and can detect major fetal abnormalities such as anencephaly and spina bifida. It can even measure the rates of blood flow through the heart valves and the large arteries of the fetus and can sometimes detect certain forms of congenital heart disease. The position of the afterbirth (*placenta*) can be determined and trouble from malposition, such as placenta praevia, anticipated. Ultrasound is also used to facilitate AMNIOCENTESIS, fetal blood sampling, CHORIONIC VILLUS SAMPLING and FETOSCOPY.

Under ultrasound control, fetal blood samples can be obtained through a fine tube, and analysed to detect coagulation disorders, infections, haemoglobin abnormalities and immunodeficiency disorders. Antibody levels in the blood can provide indications of infections such as rubella and toxoplasmosis. Biopsies can be taken for pathological examination. Exchange blood transfusion in rhesus disease can be done in the UTERUS, drug treatment given, and even certain forms of surgery performed – all under ultrasound visualization.

## Urinary problems

The commonest bladder disorder is CYSTITIS – an infection more frequent in women than in men because of readier access of organisms by way of the much shorter urethra – the tube that carries urine from the bladder to the exterior.

Involuntary urination (INCONTINENCE) is another common bladder problem. It takes various forms, the most frequent in adults being *stress incontinence* in which a small quantity of urine is passed whenever the pressure within the abdomen is suddenly increased, as in coughing or laughing.

**Excessive urination**

Production of excessive quantities of urine, or *polyuria*, may simply be due to the excessive intake of fluid, but it is commonly a sign of diseases such as diabetes mellitus, diabetes insipidus or certain diseases of the kidney, known as *salt-losing* states. Excessive urine output also occurs when oedema from any cause is treated with diuretic drugs to get rid of the excess fluid accumulated in the tissues of the body.

Excessive urination should be distinguished from over-frequent passage of small quantities of urine, as may occur in bladder infections (cystitis).

**Painful urination**
Discomfort or pain on urination, usually described as 'burning' or 'scalding', is called *dysuria*. This is often associated with difficulty in starting or a sense of incomplete emptying with a desire to continue. Painful urination is most commonly caused by bladder infection (*cystitis*), but may be due to urethritis, candidiasis of the vulva, bladder polyps, bladder cancer, stone in the bladder, or the passage of blood clots or small urinary stones. Even highly concentrated urine, as may occur in fever or excessive fluid loss in sweat, may cause discomfort.

**Urine retention**
Inability to urinate is rare in women. Retention of urine may, however, be due to a nerve disorder. This may be a transient effect on bladder control, induced by a surgical operation, a general or spinal anaesthetic, or the use of drugs which act on the bladder or the urinary sphincters; or it may arise from actual organic disease of the spinal cord or of the nerves supplying the bladder.

Urinary retention may also be due to psychological causes or may result from narrowing of the urethra from infection or pressure from uterine fibroids, or obstruction from cancer.

## Uterus

The womb or uterus is a hollow, pear-shaped organ about 8 cm long before childbirth and larger after. It has a thick, muscular wall and lies between the bladder and the rectum supported by ligaments. The lower part, the cervix, protrudes into the VAGINA.

The inner lining, the endometrium, is soft and velvety and contains many blood vessels and mucous glands. This lining changes considerably in the course of the menstrual cycle and much of it is cast off during menstruation. The two FALLOPIAN TUBES emerge at the upper, front end of the uterus, on either side.

Congenital abnormalities of the uterus affect about one woman in a hundred. Most of these are minor and unimportant, but sometimes the uterus is absent, doubled, or divided into two separate halves by a partition. Infections of the lining of the uterus may follow trauma, as in attempts at illegal abortion, or childbirth. Cervicitis may be caused by gonorrhoea, syphilis or a chlamydial or herpes infection (see SEXUALLY TRANSMITTED DISEASES). CERVICAL EROSION is a misnomer, is common and is usually unimportant.

Functional disorders of the lining of the uterus are mostly menstrual disorders of endocrine origin. Overgrowth and atrophy are common as is the growth of areas of uterine lining (*endometrium*) elsewhere in the abdomen (ENDOMETRIOSIS). See also HYSTERECTOMY, UTERUS DISPLACEMENT (PROLAPSE), UTERUS CANCER, UTERUS FIBROIDS, UTERUS RETROVERSION.

## Uterus cancer

Cancer of the lining of the UTERUS (*endometrium*) occurs most often in women between the ages of 50 and 70, and is commoner in those who have not had children. It affects mostly those who have high blood levels of oestrogen. It is much less common than cancer of the neck of the uterus (*cervix*). The first sign is usually irregular bleeding from the vagina or a blood-stained discharge. A DILATATION AND CURETTAGE (D and C) is necessary for diagnosis, and if the diagnosis has been made reasonably early and HYSTERECTOMY is performed, the outlook is usually excellent.

Cancer of the cervix is the second most common cancer in women, after BREAST CANCER. After falling steadily for many years, the incidence and mortality have now started to rise steeply, in young women in Britain. It is a common cause of death in women and is becoming commoner. Half of all cancers of the female reproductive system are in the cervix.

The disease is most likely to occur in women with a history of sexually transmitted disease, especially genital warts, women who have had many sexual partners, or whose sexual partner has genital warts, women who smoke heavily, who became pregnant at an early age and who have had three or more pregnancies. It is commonly symptomless until advanced and may cause no symptoms at all before reaching an incurable stage. Sometimes there is bleeding between periods or following sexual intercourse, but there are no dramatic early signs. Pain and general upset are rare until a late stage.

For these reasons, cancer of the cervix has to be looked for. Cervical smear screening for the pre-cancerous stage, should, ideally, be done on all women. Practical considerations dictate some restrictions, but ideally, all women should have the test at least every five years, or more often if abnormalities are found or if they are especially at risk.

Fully established cancer is difficult to treat successfully and there is no firm agreement on whether surgery or radiotherapy is best. Early cancer is commonly treated by surgery. Radiotherapy can be used at any stage. The curability depends on the extent of spread at the time of diagnosis. Early cancer, confined to the cervix, offers an excellent prognosis, with a cure rate of over 85%. But if there has been spread to the VAGINA and surrounding tissues, the cure rate drops to about 50%. Extensive spread to the organs of the pelvis and remote spread to other parts of the body, has a very poor outlook. In only about 10% of such cases is the patient still alive five years later.

## Uterus displacement (prolapse)

The UTERUS is held in position by supporting ligaments attached to the pelvis. These can be stretched and permanently lengthened during pregnancy, especially by repeated pregnancies, and this may allow the uterus to telescope down into the VAGINA (*first degree prolapse*) or even to protrude beyond the vaginal opening (*second degree*). In a third degree prolapse the whole UTERUS remains outside and the surface becomes dried, whitened and thickened.

Prolapse of the uterus is often accompanied by an unpleasant feeling of lack of support or of 'something coming down'. In descending, the uterus turns the vagina outside-in and displaces the back wall of the bladder, which is immediately in front of the vaginal wall. This leads to urinary problems including INCONTINENCE and infection.

Prolapse of the uterus is treated by surgical strengthening

of the supporting structures or, in severe cases, by removal of the UTERUS (HYSTERECTOMY). Sometimes a ring pessary can be used to keep the UTERUS in position.

## Uterus fibroids

Tumours of the body of the UTERUS are common and most of them are benign i.e., not cancers. The commonest tumours are fibroids (*leiomyomas*), which affect 10% of women of reproductive age. They are benign growths of smooth muscle and fibrous tissue, of widely varying size, which may be symptomless or may cause abnormal bleeding. Large fibroids may have local pressure effects on other organs and may interfere with pregnancy, labour or delivery. Fibroids causing trouble can be removed. In severe cases it may be best to remove the uterus (see HYSTERECTOMY).

## Uterus lining dispersion

See ENDOMETRIOSIS.

## Uterus lining inflammation

See ENDOMETRITIS.

## Uterus retroversion

The UTERUS normally lies inclined forward, at a steep angle to the backward direction of the VAGINA. A retroverted UTERUS is one which inclines in a more backward direction so that it is directly in line with the vagina, or even bent a little backwards. Formerly most of the problems which beset women, gynaecological and otherwise, were attributed to retroversion of the UTERUS, but these myths have now been dispelled and the 20% or so of women whose wombs are retroverted are now considered entirely normal.

If symptoms occur in the presence of retroversion, it is possible that they are caused by a condition which is also causing retroversion. In such a case, full investigation is necessary and the cause, if any, should be corrected.

# V

## Vagina

This is a muscular tube, 7–10 cm along its front wall and 12–15 cm along its rear wall. It is lined with a thin layer called a mucous membrane. Normally, the front and rear walls are in contact. The vagina slopes upwards and backwards. The neck of the UTERUS (*cervix*) protrudes well into the upper end of the vagina and there is a deep cul-de-sac, called the fornix, around it.

The vagina is supported by the muscles of the floor of the pelvis and these can tighten firmly around the entrance. Further up, the vagina stretches easily. The walls of the vagina are normally moist and covered with a creamy material consisting of mucoid secretions from the cervix, cast-off cells from the lining, lactic acid and many bacteria. This is normal and not a VAGINAL DISCHARGE.

During sexual excitement, the vaginal blood vessels become engorged and the lining gets thicker and hot. The upper part widens and the mucus cells in the lining mucous membrane increase their output. During orgasm, the muscles around the vagina tighten repeatedly.

## Vaginal bleeding (non-menstrual)

Bleeding originating in the vagina itself is uncommon, but may occur after forceful sexual intercourse. The real importance of vaginal bleeding is that bleeding, other than menstrual bleeding, may indicate cancer of the neck of the UTERUS (*cervix*), cancer of the lining of the uterus (*endometrium*) or ENDOMETRIOSIS. Vaginal bleeding after the menopause is a particularly important sign, which should never be ignored, but hormonal treatment, which combines progesterone with oestrogen, will cause vaginal bleeding. The contraceptive pill can cause occasional unexpected 'spotting' with blood and this may suggest that the dosage is incorrect.

Non-menstrual bleeding may also be due to soft polyps attached to the cervix, to inflammation of the cervix (*cervicitis*) or to the so-called CERVICAL EROSION. *Erosion* is actually due to spread of uterine lining to the outer surface of the cervix and bleeding from this cause is most likely after intercourse.

Vaginal bleeding in early pregnancy may indicate a threatened MISCARRIAGE. Later in pregnancy, bleeding may indicate separation of the placenta or the condition of placenta praevia in which the placenta lies over the outlet of the uterus.

## Vaginal discharge

This is one of the commonest of women's complaints. Some degree of 'discharge' is universal and normal, the material merely being the essential mucus which is secreted by glands in the uterus and cervix and by a watery fluid that passes through the walls of the vagina from the surrounding tissues. The amount of this physiological discharge varies with the stage in the menstrual cycle and tends to be greater during pregnancy. Increased secretion is also normal in states of sexual interest or excitement.

Abnormal vaginal discharge is most commonly caused by thrush (*candidiasis*) or other yeast fungi such as monilia, much less often by infection with the *Trichomonas vaginalis* organism (*trichomoniasis*).

Vaginal trichomoniasis is fairly easily treated with Flagyl (metronidazole) and this is effective so long as the sexual partner is also treated. Vaginal THRUSH is more stubborn. The infection is encouraged by pregnancy, diabetes, antibiotics and immunosuppressive drugs or conditions and aggravated by sexual intercourse, tight clothing such as jeans, nylon underwear, poor hygiene, tampons, vaginal deodorants and other sprays, and bubble baths. Contrary to the widespread belief, the oral contraceptive pill, especially the modern low-dosage pill, does not encourage thrush.

Vaginal discharge from thrush is usually treated with long-term vaginal pessaries of an anti-fungal drug, such as miconazole, inserted daily for up to six weeks. Some experts find that pessaries used twice a week for about three months, followed by once a week usage for about nine months, is effective. Less persistent treatment seems to result in recurrence, in most cases. There has been considerable success with more recent single-dose oral anti-fungal agents and these have become popular.

Vaginal discharge is sometimes caused by a forgotten tampon which has been pushed up into the cul de sac (*fornix*) behind the cervix. Occasionally a gynaecological pessary may also be left *in situ* and forgotten.

## Vaginal dryness

This is a common problem after the menopause and can lead to serious difficulties with sexual intercourse. The dryness is caused by the loss of oestrogen hormones. This loss leads to a degree of atrophy of the lining of the VAGINA and a reduction in its ability to transfer fluid through from the surrounding tissues. The condition can be greatly helped by the use of vaginal oestrogen creams (oestriol, marketed as Ortho-gynest or Ovestin) but persistent vaginal dryness after the menopause suggests that HORMONE REPLACEMENT THERAPY (HRT) may be a good idea.

## Vaginal odour

Probably the commonest cause of this is *Gardnerella vaginalis* infection. This is a very common infection of the VAGINA which produces a thin vaginal discharge with a characteristic 'fishy' odour especially in the presence of a mild alkali, such as toilet soap. There are no other symptoms, but the organism, and the odour, can be sexually transmitted to the partner. The infection tends to be stubborn, but responds well to treatment with the drug Flagyl (metronidazole).

## Varicose veins

Twisted, expanded and distorted veins, usually occurring in the legs, but sometimes at the lower end of the gullet (*oesophagus*). Varicose veins of the legs are a misery and an embarrassment to millions, causing much distress by their unsightly appearance and the associated symptoms. Women, especially, are the victims of varicose veins and are affected more often, and more severely, than men.

Varicosity means stagnation of blood flow, poor oxygenation and nutrition to the surrounding tissues and the accumulation of metabolites which would normally be washed away and diluted by a free blood flow. The result is aching and tiredness in the legs, persistent swelling of the ankles, brownish-blue discoloration of the skin, a tendency to ulceration after minor injury and, rarely, dangerous bleeding from a ruptured vein.

The force of the heartbeat, which maintains the arterial pressure and drives the blood to all parts of the body, is almost expended by the time the blood has passed through the capillaries and reached the veins. So blood flow in the veins is passive and the pressure is very low, and this is reflected in the structure of the veins, which are thin-walled and collapse easily. Arteries have thick, elastic walls and never collapse, even when empty.

Blood returning from the head, neck and upper chest is assisted by gravity, but blood from the lower part of the body, especially the legs, has to fight gravity. A series of one-way valves in the veins allows the blood to move only in the direction of the heart, and any compression of the veins forces the column of blood to move in this direction. This external pressure is supplied by the changing shape of adjacent muscles as they contract. In the legs, most of the vein pumping is done by the calf muscles when they are contracting to extend the ankle. Interestingly, the symptoms of varicose veins are often relieved by walking.

The weight of the column of blood from the heart to the ankles is considerable and would be sufficient to cause stretching and bulging, were the veins not adequately supported by surrounding tissue. Fortunately, when all is as it should be, this heavy column of blood is broken up into sections by the valves, and its weight distributed.

The deep veins of the leg, which are large enough to carry all the returning blood, lie among the leg muscles and form an effective pump. The surface, or superficial, veins, however, lie just under the skin, are less well supported and do not receive the same all-round compressive force. These surface veins join the main deep veins up in the groin, but, at various levels in the legs, they also have cross connections to the deep veins, called the perforating veins. These, too, contain valves allowing one-way movement of blood from the superficial to the deep veins.

If the valves in the perforating veins do not close properly on back pressure, the muscle pump pressure in the deep veins is transferred to the less well-supported surface veins and the result is stretching. Once valves become leaky (*incompetent*), varicosity is inevitable. It is not known whether the primary problem is undue distensibility of the veins, so that the valves become incompetent, or whether the basis is constitutionally incompetent valves. Varicose veins tend to run in families and there is certainly a genetic tendency to one or the other of these causes – perhaps both. Other factors contribute – obesity, insufficient exercise, pregnancy, prolonged standing and local constriction from underwear elastic or garters.

Uniform, overall support, with no local tourniquet effect, can, on the other hand, be very helpful in the management of varicose veins of the legs. Well-designed and properly selected elastic stockings (*compression hosiery*) prevent stagnation, divert the blood into the deep veins where the muscle pump works better, prevent the reflux of blood from the deep veins and generally keep the blood flowing as it should. Stagnation is abolished, tissue nutrition improved, symptoms relieved. Even established varicose ulcers have been known to heal.

The compression should be greater at the ankle than at the thigh and should be graded along the leg. This requirement is now acknowledged by manufacturers and incorporated into the design of their products.

If compression hosiery fails, varicose veins may have to be closed off by injection of a clotting solution, or even removed altogether by the operation of stripping.

## Virginity

The state of a person who has never had sexual intercourse. Properly, the term is applied to a girl or woman.

The notion that the only physical sign of virginity is an intact HYMEN can be misleading. Hymens vary considerably in thickness, extent and rigidity and in some cases may stretch, without tearing, during sexual intercourse. In addition, a hymen may be torn in the course of an accident or fall involving trauma to the area. In most cases, however, the hymen is torn during the first sexual penetration.

In some parts of the world, men continue to make much of the importance of virginity in those they wish to marry, and women are still persecuted for the effects of submitting to male importunity. Real social equality demands that such attitudes should either be reciprocal or, more realistically, abandoned.

## Virilism

The state of masculinization in the female. Virilism is caused by an excess of certain male sex hormones (*androsterones*). This has several major effects on the female. There is:

- increased growth of body hair in the male distribution pattern

- balding at the temples
- reduction or cessation of the menstrual periods
- loss of the characteristically female fat deposits around the hips
- enlargement of the clitoris
- an increase in the development of the arm and shoulder muscles
- acne
- deepening of the voice due to enlargement of the voice box (*larynx*)

Virilization occurs in certain diseased states in which the adrenal glands and, to a lesser extent, the ovaries, secrete excess of the normal male hormones, the androsterones. This may occur in tumours of the adrenal glands or ovaries, either benign or malignant, or in the condition of congenital adrenal hyperplasia. This condition results from a genetic defect which interferes with the synthesis of cortisol. The resulting low cortisol levels prompt the pituitary to produce increased quantities of adrenocorticotrophic hormone (ACTH). But ACTH stimulates production of male sex hormones as well as corticosteroids and, since the latter cannot be produced, the result is a rise, to abnormal levels, of the androsterones. These are converted, in the body, to the powerful male sex hormone testosterone which is the cause of the virilization.

The treatment of virilism is to deal with the cause.

## Vulva

The female external genitalia, comprising the pad of fat over the pubic bone (*mons pubis*), the two pairs of LABIA (*labia majora* and *labia minora*), the area between the labia minora, and the entrance to the VAGINA (*introitus*).

## Vulval disorders

Because of the proximity to the anus, the vulva are always contaminated with organisms of many types. Nevertheless, inflammation (*vulvitis*) is usually controlled by natural local resistance. Vulvitis most commonly results from genital HER-PES or THRUSH (*candidiasis*), especially in diabetics, but occurs also from oestrogen deficiency, or contact allergies to soaps, deodorants or traces of 'biological' washing powder remaining on underwear after washing. The vulva may be the site of a primary sore (*chancre*) in syphilis. Bartholinitis is inflammation of the BARTHOLIN'S GLANDS which lie between the opening of the vagina and the labia minora. Bartholinitis may proceed to abscess formation and this may require surgical opening. Vulvovaginitis is vulvitis associated with inflammation in the vagina, and this is usually caused by candidiasis or trichomoniasis.

# W

## Warning signs

There are several well-recognized signs which should be known to all as they may give early warning of cancer or other serious disease. They should always be reported. The warning signs are:

- a new, changed or persisting cough
- coughing blood
- black stools or rectal bleeding
- any persistent change in the bowel habit
- indigestion coming on for the first time in later life
- difficulty in swallowing
- vomiting blood
- blood in the urine
- any obvious change in a coloured skin spot, mole or wart
- any sore that fails to heal in a month
- hoarseness or loss of voice, without obvious cause
- unexplained weight loss
- postmenopausal vaginal bleeding

## Weight problems

Weight loss is the result of a dietary calorie intake which is smaller than the calorie expenditure. This may be the result of a deliberate, weight-losing policy in the interests of health, an abnormal reduction in food intake as in ANOREXIA NERVOSA or DEPRESSION, or unavoidable starvation. Weight loss, from excess of tissue breakdown (*catabolism*) over build up (*anabolism*), is also a feature of many diseases, particularly thyroid overactivity, cancer, tuberculosis and diabetes. Reduced calorie intake may also result from malabsorption disorders or from intestinal disorder such as persistent vomiting or diarrhoea.

Unexplained weight loss is one of the warning signs of possible serious disease and should never be disregarded.

**Weight reduction**

All dietary intake in excess of the energy requirements is converted to fat. This is stored mainly under the skin, but also inside the abdomen. So a big tummy is due to fat both inside and outside the abdominal wall. Human fat is an oily liquid at body temperature and it is helpful to think of the surplus fat store as being like oil in a tank. Reducing weight has nothing to do with getting rid of solid tissue; it is simply a matter of using up this oil faster than it accumulates. If you eat more than you need, the level of oil will rise. If you eat less than you need to fuel your energy expenditure (keeping warm, walking, moving about, etc) the level in the tank will drop and you will get thinner. It is as simple as that.

Reduced calorie intake is a far more efficient way of reducing weight than taking exercise. But regular exercise is an essential part of the process of weight reduction. Contrary to expectation, exercise helps to limit food intake. Weight cannot, however, be lost, in health, without reducing intake, so suffering and hunger are inevitable. New, smaller, eating habits must be established. 'Crash' diets, fad diets, or those involving non-nutritious food substitutes, as widely advertised on TV, are generally a waste of time, as they do not get at the basic requirement to amend a long-sustained habit of putting too much in your mouth. The only effective way to achieve permanent weight reduction must also be long-sustained. For this reason, would-be weight reducers who spend money on health farms, proprietary diets, books and magazines on dieting, and expensive exercising equipment are dodging the real issue.

The kind of food taken is less important than the quantity, but a diet should, in addition to being of small quantity, be well balanced with plenty of vegetable roughage and fruit, a moderate intake of protein – preferably from fish and poultry – and a minimum of fat and dairy products. It should contain no butter or margarine and milk should be skimmed. Above all, it must be low in quantity.

## Wife battering

It is difficult to decide whether this is becoming more common or merely more conspicuous. It is clear that this is not a minor and isolated phenomenon and that it spreads across all the socio-economic groups. Since the proportion of cases reported cannot be determined, hard statistics are not available, but estimates, based on known data, suggest that up to 1% of women living with men are abused in this way.

There is evidence that wife batterers are often the product of homes in which the mother was beaten by the father. They are, also, often men of a 'macho' disposition, who, lacking the intellectual and cultural resources to resolve life problems, instinctively turn to physical aggression. Such men, suitably mated, may form reasonably stable, if stormy, relationships. Unfortunately, battered wives are often inadequate, reserved, anxious, depressed and timid, with a low sense of their own value and a high level of dependence on others. Their own parents were often unable to express affection and inclined to encourage submissiveness. Such women may find themselves in a trap – desperately unhappy, but unable to bring themselves to leave the man and face the terrors of the unknown.

The patterns of domestic violence against women are clear. Starting with quarrels and sustained verbal abuse, prompted by any of the common causes of domestic discord, the process escalates to an initial physical assault which is usually minor – perhaps an aggressive shove – then a slap or a punch. Most affected women report that they expected the assaults to stop at that point, but study of case histories shows that the common pattern is one of increasing levels of violence with a lowering of the provocation needed to bring on an attack. Attempts on the part of the woman to defend herself may seem to the man to be a threat to his authority and to justify his anger. Such women are in real danger of serious injury, especially if alcohol further diminishes the man's inhibitions.

Numerous case reports show that the pattern is often cyclical, episodes of violence being followed by periods of remorse, but with a steady escalation to ever more violent and savage assault, sometimes culminating in murder. No woman, whatever her circumstances, should submit silently to physical abuse. Tragically, for many, the alternatives – economic loss, social humiliation, official prying – may seem even worse. The threat of legal action may be salutary – and wife beaters should be reminded that the courts are taking an ever more serious view of the problem. But even if the offender goes to prison, the greater punishment may still be suffered by the woman.

## Withdrawal bleeding

Bleeding from the lining of the UTERUS caused by a sudden drop in the blood levels of the female sex hormones progesterone or oestrogen. This occurs naturally in menstruation, and at the end of each cycle of use of the oral contraceptive pill, but may also be a feature of cessation of any treatment with these hormones, for any purpose.

## Womb

See UTERUS.

## Womb removal

See HYSTERECTOMY.

# X

## Xanthelasma

This is deposit of cholesterol in the skin of the eyelids, above and below the inner corner of the eye, which causes unsightly, raised, yellow plaques. These become larger and increasingly conspicuous with time. Xanthelasma is sometimes, but not always, associated with raised blood cholesterol, but its presence justifies a blood check as it is commonly present in the dangerous condition of familial hypercholesterolaemia.

Treatment, for cosmetic reasons, is easy, as the lid skin is usually lax and the plaques can easily be removed. Recurrence is, however, common.

# INDEX

# COLLINS POCKET REFERENCE

*Other titles in the Pocket Reference series:*

## Prescription Drugs
Clear, uncomplicated explanations of prescription
drugs and their actions

## Etiquette
A practical guide to what is and what is not
acceptable and expected in modern society

## Speaking in Public
A guide to speaking with confidence,
whatever the occasion

## Ready Reference
A fascinating source of information on measurements,
symbols, codes and abbreviations

## Weddings
An invaluable guide to all wedding arrangements,
from the engagement to the honeymoon

## Card Games
A guide to the rules and strategies of play
for a wide selection of card games

*(All titles £4.99)*